The Art of REinvention:

Transforming Brushstrokes into a Living Masterpiece

By
Tanya R. Bankston, MA, LLPC
Change Doula
REinvention Strategist

Published by Greater Heights Coaching & Professional Development LLC.

The Art of Reinvention
Copyright © 2018 by Tanya R. Bankston

ISBN-13: 978-0-9993854-1-8

Unless otherwise noted, all scriptures are derived from the King James Version Bible.

Cover design by www.goonwrite.com
Interior design by Doris AC Johnson
Edited by Doris AC Johnson
Publishing Consultant: Andre'a T Robinson Inside My Mind Publishing

Printed in the United States of America

FOREWORD

For human beings to thrive and not just survive, we must have a grasp of who we are and our place in the larger world around us. We achieve this both on an individual journey of discovery and through connection to kindred spirits we encounter along the way. One of the greatest barriers to healing is isolation because when we live alone in our pain, we lack the critical element of perspective – an accurate view of the bigger picture and a heartfelt understanding that…this too shall pass. Tanya Bankston has done more than written a book. She has issued an invitation to all those women who suffer alone in the darkness of their pain and shame, to come forward into the light. With insight and striking vulnerability, she sacrificially offers the reader her own painful story of tragedy and victory as a warm hand of friendship, willing to guide others towards their own healing. My hope is that each person who reads this will find the courage to, in Tanya's words, *"Walk with their head held high, exchanging beauty for ashes, the oil of joy for mourning and the garment of praise for the spirit of heaviness."*

Terry D. McGlasson, Ph.D., Associate Professor of Counseling – Central Michigan University

ENDORSEMENTS

"Mrs. Tanya Bankston (Coach T) shares her personal vivid heartfelt story of personal pain as it relates to rejection and low self-esteem. Her story mirrors the journey of so many women. Tanya compassionately advocates for women who has yet gained the strength or the courage to share their tragic pain of emotional, sexual, and psychological abuse. Tanya freely and honestly displays passion and determination to destroy the messages that were designed to massacre her vision, purpose and destiny. One of the most compelling aspects of this book is her specific methodology that was birthed from her journey for authentic healing. The words that begin with RE provides for the reader an opportunity to start again. Restoration, Rejuvenation, Renew, Recharge, Recreate, Refocus, Realignment, Revive, Reflection, Reconnection, Rejoice, Revitalized, Reposition, Reinvention, and Redeemed are words that speak life into the readers, traumatic situation and perspective. The book offers a road map for self-discovery and reconstruction of the mindset that has been plagued with self-destruction and self-pity. Tanya promotes the power of God's word for her personal restoration and as a declaration for woman who suffers in silence. Tanya challenges the reader to take action! The Art of REinvention is a Masterpiece!"

Dr. Christal Eason, PhD, LMSW, Author, Speaker, Coach

"Tanya Bankston has done more than written a book. She has issued an invitation to all those women who suffer alone in the darkness of their pain and shame, to come forward into the light."

Terry D. McGlasson, Ph.D., *Associate Professor of Counseling –*
Central Michigan University
"The Art of REinvention: Transforming Life Challenges into a Living
Masterpiece is a wonderful companion for us if we are in the midst of
experiencing emotional pain with the desire to heal.

This book is an awesome companion for us who are on the mend. For
us who have crossed the threshold and are now able to reflect and
marvel at our REinvention. Tanya's heart reaches us, as she lovingly
and courageously shares the pieces of her heart, mind, soul and Spirit.
She connects with us, as we journal among the powerful expressions,
she creatively transfers from mind to hand to pen to paper. This book
is one where we may truly feel at one with ourselves...with Sisterhood.
Thank You, Tanya, BeautifulSpiritSisterFriend for loving us to
share."

Anita C Powell, *Metaphysical Life Coach/Teacher*
Engai Poetry & Music Publishing TAP N2U

"I stand in awe of Coach Tanya's vulnerability, transparency,
honesty, and courage to tell her the truth, stand in her truth and
encourage other women to do the same. Not only is she sharing her
story but teaching us how to transcend and move beyond the pain of
the past; and use the lessons we have learned to redefine who we are
and who we have the power to be. The Art of REinvention is a
Masterpiece."

Sister2Sister Inspirational Network CEO, **Tamera J. Moore,**
LLPC

"If you are seeking to be REstored, to be REjuvenated, and to be Renewed, "The Art of REinvention" is the book for you. Tanya Bankston's story is one of how her innocence was shattered and it took decades for her to understand the effects that it would have on her life. This book strategically reels you in through your feelings of familiarity. It unlocks places in the heart that have been securely locked away for years but gives you a sense of relief while relating to every word. The author takes you on a path of revitalizing your spirit after being broken, from sexual abuse, rejection and low self-esteem. It reaches down to your very core and offers hope for living a life of healing and self-love. What will you gain from reading "The Art of REinvention?" You will learn that in your time of darkness you can realign your life and unveil the thing you have carried so deeply and for so long. You will learn how to reinvent yourself and shine brightly like the beautiful diamond that you are. The Art of REinvention is an excellent read. I recommend this book, because it gives you the courage to recognize your own insecurities and helps define how!"

Denise Cochran, Certified Life Coach
Best-Selling Author of *"Fearless Women Rock: Courageous Women Find Strength During The Storm."*

"I was recently asked to review a book written by one of my former students, Tanya Bankston. Her compelling tale is one of personal change and redemption entitled "The Art of REInvention." This clever title reminded me of a former topic of this newsletter publication "The Price of Change". In our former communication, we pointed out that all change brings with it two somewhat and, perhaps, paralyzing side effects: fear and a sense of loss. What is there to fear in a promising job opportunity or an exciting new relationship? While, perhaps the

new career opportunity will be disappointing. Maybe the new guy (or woman) turns out to be a jerk. Any change has the potential to backfire on us. What is there to lose in change? First and foremost, there is almost certainly a loss of security. Even if we hate our current job or relationship partnership, at least we have come to understand and accept it. It is said that if a farmer or horseman leads his horses out of a burning barn, he must secure them somehow or they, in fear, will run back into the burning barn. The barn is their source of security and, in a panic, the terrified animal will run back to their source of comfort and security. Clearly, however majestic the stallion or mare may be, they aren't very smart. But we aren't horses. And yet, there are times when we may "run back into the barn" out of fear or a sense of loss. What's the solution? Act courageously, recognizing that courage involves action in the face of fear; not in the absence of it. So, my former student, Tanya, showed great courage in the telling of her story. She shared her pain in the hope that her tale will allow others to learn and benefit from it. It was also an act of "reinvention" for her in order to move forward positively in her life. I admire her greatly for that bravery. Homework: What "barns" have you returned to in your life? What changes for the better are you avoiding in exchange for the security of mediocrity? Courage!"

Dr. John Farrar, PhD, LPD
Author of *The Snowman Theory* http://snowmantherapy.com/tbf-theory/and dump the *Neanderthal; Choose your Prime Mate*

"I just finished reading your incredibly heart-breaking/heart-healing, hopeful book. You are a gifted, creative writer. It is evident that this book was truly written from the inner core of your soul. No child should have to endure your experience nor should any woman be subjected to those so vividly related in your book. I admire your

DEDICATION

This book is dedicated to all the women who have shared their story of pain with me in confidence, and the many women who have never shared their story with anyone. Thank you for sharing your stories with me, making it clear that my secret tears were not in vain. My unique story is one that is common in human existence.

I have a testimony, and it needs to be shared. There is healing…there is deliverance…and there is Joy after the *mourning*.

PREFACE

This is a book of emotional healing. Initially, when I started writing, it appeared as a "tell all" of my dirty little secrets. These dirty secrets were intimate details of events that I used to be ashamed of, and struggled for years to hide, deny and forget.

I have found these incidents to be the subject of conversations with other women across the country. Although, each story has a unique set of circumstances, these discussions often share the same theme. They include incidents of sexual molestation, rape, abortion, children born out of wedlock, the pain associated with divorce, physical/mental/verbal/sexual abuse, and self-esteem/self-image issues.

The only difference between me and some of the women that I speak to in my private encounters is the decision that I made to discontinue carrying the shame, guilt, and pain like an expensive designer handbag that I was afraid to place down.

This book is about sharing parts of my life in a way that helped me bring closure to painful experiences in my past and move beyond those painful memories.

I call these challenging experiences, "Brushstrokes." In life, we cannot connect all the dots perfectly, color in the lines, or draw without erasing. Paint splatters, and spills make stains. We cannot scrap the picture, which is the canvas of our life, and begin again, so what do we do? The Art of REinvention discusses the process of transforming Brushstrokes, or life challenges that could have broken, and/or destroyed us into a "Living Masterpiece." I share tips on how to weave those zany, "color outside of the line" life experiences into your Masterpiece based on your declaration of how you define your life as artwork. This is my story of what I went through, what I learned, and how I recovered. You may not have the desire or courage to share your Brushstrokes with the world, but you can free yourself from the prison of the pain and declare your own Living Masterpiece. You can paint a different picture and maintain control of your paintbrush!

INTRODUCTION

The Art of REinvention is more than a rebuilding. So why REinvention as art or art form? Why the CAPITAL letters for RE?

First, I describe REinvention as an art form because it takes special skill, and technique to go through life's challenges and learn to GROW through them rather than to go through them. In fact, it takes resilience to REcover from some of life's greatest challenges. REsilience is the capacity to recover quickly from difficulties, toughness. The ability of a substance or object to spring back into shape; elasticity. I believe some people are born with a great capacity of resilience and others can learn to be more resilient through coping strategies. Personally, it is my belief that I have been blessed with both.

Now, why the CAPITAL RE?

"Re" means again or "again and again" to indicate repetition, or with the meaning "back" or "backward." I use it as in capital letters to draw attention to the process. The Art of REinvention is more than a rebuilding. A rebuilding takes in consideration many of the old working parts combined with the new parts. REinvention takes into consideration the process of utilizing all the old parts and REinventing them! None of the old parts are discarded. Our lives are just like that...the old parts are not discarded. We can decide to learn from past mistakes, and challenges, or we can succumb to them.

I have learned there is a reason and purpose for every circumstance in life. We often don't understand God's reason until long after we have experienced the test or trial. I have come to believe that growing through tests and trials is for the benefit of a testimony to share with others.

As a matter of fact, I am convinced this is the case! Honestly, this hasn't always been my belief and I have suffered in silence for many years with various struggles because I was too afraid to share my testimony. My fear kept me isolated, ashamed, and embarrassed about enduring life events that other people have endured and overcame.

Let's start by clarifying some terms in the context of how I use them.

Art:

The expression or application of human creative skill and imagination, typically in a visual form such as painting, sculpture, producing works to be appreciated primarily for their beauty or emotional power. (Google) Art is personalized, it's unique, and it's self-expressive. How one person defines art may be interpreted as garbage, or junk by another person. Art is relative to the person viewing the art.

The type of art created is going to determine some of the basic tools used to express it. For example, a painter uses brushes, canvas, paints, easel, pencils, etc. A dancer uses music, coordination, choreography, rhythm, etc. and the art is poetry in motion. A writer or speaker will use nouns, verbs, hyperboles, adjectives, prose, etc. to create visual imagery in the mind of the reader or listening audience.

Masterpiece:

A work of outstanding artistry, skill, or workmanship. (Google) I would like to add that raw materials are used in the expression of art...this book is about transforming your raw materials (talents, skills, experiences, challenges, mishaps, mess ups, screw ups, blunders, etc. ok you get the picture). We each start with raw materials, but it is the transformation of those raw materials that is the focus of my masterpiece that you are reading. As you take this journey, I would like for you to focus on three concepts.

First, if you can relate because you have been through a similar situation, look at the points that are common themes in your story. We tend to repeat life themes until we become aware of them, or our need to change, and take interventive measures to change our behavior.

This will have a compatible section in the book entitled: **Relate.** Use the **Relate** section to detail your account of the hurtful experience. The second concept is the **Recover** section of the experience. In this section detail your thoughts, emotions, and other points of importance to help you in the recovery process. It is one thing to go through an incident, it is another concept to recover from the experience and mature past the experience. The final concept to take into consideration is the section entitled: **Release.** This is the section where you give a detailed account of your emotions and look for healthy methods to release the pain. Just as there are many unhealthy ways of dealing with the pain, such as excessive use/abuse of alcohol, the use and abuse of both prescription/illegal drugs, over-eating, compulsive shopping, and gambling; there are many techniques to develop healthy habits for healing. Some examples of healthy options can include mental health therapy, journaling, twelve step programs, and physical exercise. Although this is a self-help book, it is for informational purposes only and does not constitute medical advice; the content is not intended to be a substitute for professional medical or therapeutic advice, diagnosis, or treatment. Always seek the advice of a physician or other qualified mental health provider with any questions you may have regarding a medical condition. Never disregard professional medical advice or delay in seeking it because of something you have read in this book. Use this book as a self-discovery tool to serve as a catalyst for transforming your brushstrokes into your living masterpiece.

Coach Tanya Bankston
Change Doula and Brushstrokes Reinvention Coach

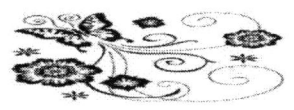

Table of Contents

FOREWORD
ENDORSEMENTS
DISCLAIMER
DEDICATION
PREFACE
INTRODUCTION
ACKNOWLEDGMENT

To my mother Kassandra E. Christopher (1952-2019):
Though the words in this manuscript made you cry, you now know
no sorrows…

ACKNOWLEDGMENTS

I want to give honor to my savior Jesus Christ for saving my life and showing me through the word of God that Restoration is possible from damaged emotions.

To Anthony and Brian, I am so honored to be your mother. I began to understand unconditional love raising you both. I have made many mistakes as a mother, but you loved me beyond my faults. Sorry about all the spankings…love you forever!

To my mom, we haven't always agreed on things, but I know you have always loved me. Thank you for the amazing love of reading and writing that set the foundation for me! Now that I am older and wiser, I understand the majority of the times we didn't agree, I wasn't ready for the truth.

To my granny, (my G-mommy) thank you for all the times we spent sharing stories, and all the wisdom that you have poured into my spirit.

To my sister Margaret and my brother Dione, thank you for loving me despite myself. Lamont, we were alike in many ways...I love and miss you baby brother.

To my aunts, Leronia and Carolyn, I love you both, and yes, I am my granny's baby daughter. Aunt Joyce, you are a special golden touch added to our family.

To Uncle Gerald, thank you for being my favorite uncle…and I forgive you for spanking me.

To My cousins Sharima, David, and Christina who knew you were onto something when you started calling me "Tyrone."

To my twin Kathy, oh my God! The last twenty-five years have

been a blast! We have prayed, laughed, cried and healed, and you have taught me to love and forgive! It has been a journey! You also taught me about the heart string connection...

My friend Vera, I love you forever. You have always believed in me; Rest in heaven until we meet again.

To my girl, Felicia...my sister to the end, thank you!

Darlene, I have mad love for you and your support!

To all my Second Ebenezer Church family, thanks for your love and support.

I love my entire Champion for Change Sisters! You know who you are! I am so blessed to have so many wonderful sisters.

A special thanks to both, Veda Sharp and Kim Nolte for mentoring me and giving me a chance when no one else would.

To my Mr. Wonderful, my husband Robert, it's amazing that the first day I met you, I didn't like you, and yet I have spent every day with you since our meeting. You are not perfect, but you are perfect for me! You have taught me to hold that mirror up to myself and check my motives. Our love makes forgiveness, Action in Practice.

1 Shining Pass the Veil of Rejection

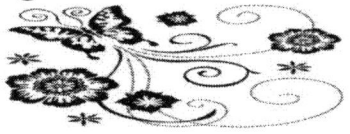

Rejection tears at the fabric of the human soul; sending a message that destroys a woman's self-esteem, self-value, and self-worth. ~ Tanya R Bankston

When I think about the fact that my life could have been aborted more than forty-nine years ago by a straightened metal clothes hanger inserted into my sixteen-year-old mother's womb, I am grateful that God…He had another plan!

I haven't always been grateful. Because my mother thought of terminating my life, I was born with a spirit of rejection looming over me. In fact, for more than half of my life, I was angry, bitter, and felt rejected. My mother gave birth to me at a time in history when teenagers were not awarded reality TV shows for getting pregnant before getting married.

One definition of rejection, as written in the Oxford English Dictionary reads: "the emotional refusal or inability to accept one's own child; the state of rejecting a child, or of being rejected by a parent." My mother was sheltered, afraid, and misinformed about sexuality. As she told me that she contemplated aborting me, feelings of rage, guilt, and shame engulfed me. I wasn't ready for her type of truth. Her blunt honesty was too much reality for my young mind and cut my heart into many pieces like a sharpened blade.

This conversation began as one of our normal mother-daughter bonding sessions but ended with my need for emotional reconstructive surgery. She meant no harm, but at sixteen years old, it led to dark thoughts swirling within me. I wondered, "Could my mother ever love me after initially rejecting me? Was I so vile and repulsive that I drove my father out of my life, too?"

I agonized mentally and wondered: "Why did God create such a hideous, creature like me?" For years I thought of myself as a hideous, ugly, black monster, unworthy of love and acceptance. Growing up, the deep root of rejection made me feel inadequate, unaccepted, and incomplete. Rejection made me feel I never fit in; that I was out of place in every setting. I always felt my presence wasn't welcome because I constantly heard messages of rejection everywhere, I went that stained my soul.

"You are too thin."

"You are so black."

"You look like that creature from the black lagoon."

"You are a pretty girl to be SO BLACK."

"Your feet are too big."

I heard these negative descriptions of myself so often that I cried all the time. I constantly felt sad and depressed because I was rejected by my peers, my father, and my mother. These messages, both internal and external, stung me to my inner core. When I look back, I marvel that I did not develop into a sadistic serial killer or die from several suicide attempts. It is obvious God had another plan.

My rejection was affirmed repeatedly until puberty knocked at my door. I was still black, and thin, but I had gained two new friends: my BREASTS.

At first, I really enjoyed having breasts. However, after some time, they started to contribute to my sense of rejection because of the unsolicited attention they brought me. I was one of the first girls in my neighborhood to develop breasts.

After that, I suddenly became popular with the guys in the neighborhood. The budding of my breasts and the curve of my hips gave me a newfound impetus to seek the acceptance and approval I craved from my newly attentive male suitors. Part of me enjoyed this new-found attention, but the other part of me understood that is was only temporary. I didn't care how temporary this attention was, it felt good to be sought after and desired.

Sadly, this attention turned harmful because I became the victim of repeated sexual abuse at the age of twelve. The first time I was molested, I followed the rules and told an adult quickly. After I told, I thought I would be protected. I thought I would be believed. I thought someone would speak up for me and comfort me. Once again, my attempt to do the right thing was rebuffed and my lifelong message of rejection was again reinforced!

The next time I was molested, I hesitated about telling an adult. I was approached by a male acquaintance of the family who asked if he could fondle my breasts if he gave me money. Although, I knew it was wrong, I felt it was okay since I didn't have a job or have a regular allowance. Twenty-five dollars seemed an appropriate sum to allow him to fondle my breasts. Here I was at the tender age of twelve negotiating a sexual deal. I rationalized doing this because I had had money, which I wanted…it was a win-win situation. This perfectly arranged deal took a nose-dive into disaster when my mother found out. That experience quickly taught me the influence of my sexuality on men, and I just wanted to capitalize on it. However, after this episode,

I hesitated to tell another adult because this man was an "adult." After this experience, a seed was planted inside me that adults could not be trusted, especially men! Because of these encounters, I believed the only type of love or physical affection I deserved involved giving away my virtue.

My innocence was shattered. I rationalized that I wasn't hurting myself, but I was very wrong. It would take me decades before I understood the true darkness and the residual effects that these types of negotiations had on me spiritually, psychologically, emotionally, and physically. The veil of shame over how I was treated cast me into a deep depression and threatened to silence my radiance and sparkle.

Just as God had other plans for me to be here, He also had a greater plan to unearth the brilliance lying dormant within me. After rededicating my life to Christ, God began to fill my spirit with words to meditate and facilitate my healing. The black veil covering me begin to lift as I meditated on the words the Holy Spirit dropped into my spirit. These words combated the spirit of Rejection and I adopted new words: Restoration, Rejuvenation, Renew, Recharge, Recreate, Refocus, Realignment, Revive, Reflection, Reconnection, Rejoice, Revitalize, Reposition, Reinvention, and Redeemed.

My lifelong feelings of inadequacy were not a message from God and as I meditated the Word of God, those dark feelings of shame, guilt, unforgiveness, and bitterness began to melt away. I began to walk with my head held high as I exchanged beauty for ashes, the oil of joy for mourning, the garment of praise for the spirit of heaviness, just as God promised in His Word. As I began to speak my truth and share my experiences with other women, I began to understand that my story of sexual abuse, shame, and guilt were not uniquely my story alone. Other women suffered the same pain and walked around covered with the same veil of darkness. My heavenly Father began to reveal how important it is for me to speak up and speak out to other women in bondage in order to shed light on the darkness of the enemy.

2009 became a year of purging past hurt.

I must be totally honest: in the beginning, it was difficult because I had experienced so much pain at the hands of men, it was almost impossible to trust God. However, as He revealed himself through His Word, I began to trust God not to hurt me. I began to believe the truth in God's power to love me and understand that everything I had gone through; every experience, both good and bad, would be used by God for a greater purpose in my life. It was at this same time God began to reveal himself to me and helped me to step outside of my comfort zone.

As I begin speaking to others about my life, I was transformed from resisting God to being REsiliant through God.

My hope for the future was REstored, and my brilliance was unearthed as I allowed God to transform my thoughts, my speech, and my actions.

Ironically at times, I still expected God to lie, but His Word promised me it's impossible for Him to lie, and I learned that His Word would not return to him void. I began to trust and understand that He is not a man therefore, He cannot lie. The more I trusted God to perform His word in my life, the more my life began to change.

I graduated from college, changed careers, got married, and I started a business. I am reminded that just as my past is not unique; the victory of transformation is also available to all. Part of my growth included stepping out of the darkness and in the limelight as I shared my story. Each time I step onto a stage, the spirit of rejection whispers thoughts of ridicule to me, a hissing reminder of my past. However, I push pass those inner voices and I encourage myself in order to share my story to free my sisters from bondage.

Women share with me constantly their similar stories of abuse, rejection, shame, and guilt. I am amazed at how the characters change, but the story is similar or identical to mine. Many of my sisters still suffer in silence and I encourage them to allow their sparkle to shine. Out of the depths of despair, rejection, guilt, and shame buried beneath the muck and mire, trampled, and discarded lying beneath the surface was a young woman whose desire was to be loved and accepted.

Today she shines, she walks in her authenticity, she is no longer afraid of rejection's sting, and she sparkles and glistens. Her worth is more valuable than rubies. She wears strength and honor as her clothing rather than the rags of rejection. She openly shares her story with hurting women to pull them up to a place of clarity and grace as the veil of rejection is lifted in their lives.

I am that woman…I am still being polished, and I am still discovering my beauty and my worth, but I will continue to shine.

The raggedy rejected pieces of my soul have been woven into a shining cloak of beauty and grace. God used every strand of thread for His Glory.

~Tanya R Bankston

R E late

In this section write a detailed response to a situation that you have been in when you felt rejected? Be sure to write as many of the facts including who the offender was, when the incident occurred, where it occurred, times, dates, etc. Use additional paper if needed. How could this situation have ended differently?

What type of signs do you see in your present life that were shaped by this experience?

What did you do at the time to notify someone else about the incident? Were you able to share the information with a friend, a relative, or a person of authority?

How could things have ended differently on a negative note?

How could things have ended differently on a positive note?

_____

_____

_____

_____

_____

_____

_____

_____

_____

_____

_____

_____

_____

_____

_____

_____

_____

_____

Did you have feelings of anger, shame, embarrassment or guilt? What did you do to help you deal with these emotions? Are you still carrying the emotions around unresolved?

R E cover

In this section, detail your thoughts, emotions, and other points of importance to help you in the recovery process...details are good! It is especially important to write down your feelings. They may include anger, disappointment, fear, rejection, shame, guilt, betrayal, etc. These strong emotions should be identified and addressed. It is important to acknowledge your feelings and release those emotions.

Write freely and use additional sheets of paper, if necessary. Be careful not to pass judgment on yourself for acknowledging your emotions. These are normal emotions, and we all experience these various emotions.

Imagine that you are having a conversation with the person who offended, violated, or rejected you. Sit them down in a chair. This is called the empty chair technique…take a chair and have a conversation with them. Say everything that you wanted to say but were too afraid, embarrassed, angry, etc. to say.

Say it! Say it loud, cry, yell, etc. just get it out in a space that is safe for you.

The good thing is they must listen while you speak without interruptions. Really get it all out!

Write about this experience after you complete the exercise.

Did this exercise evoke feelings of sadness, empowerment, anger, etc.? Please write your response in detail. Understand that as you write there is a degree of release associated with journaling the experience. It is a good idea to share your thoughts and emotions with a trusted friend, relative, or licensed mental health professional, such as a social worker, mental health therapist, or licensed counselor.

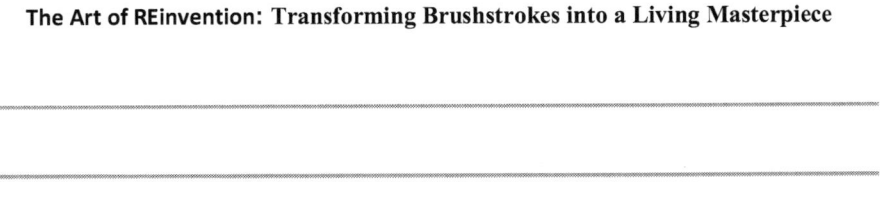

RElease

In this section, let's review some healthy techniques to release those emotions towards the person who offended or harmed you.

Just as there are many unhealthy ways of dealing with the pain, such as excessive use of alcohol, the use and abuse of prescribed and illegal drugs, overeating, compulsive shopping, and gambling; there are many techniques that can be used to develop healthy habits for healing.

Some examples of healing options can include mental health therapy, twelve steps programs, journaling, and exercise (just to name a few). This journey will include exercises, and resourceful information to aid you in moving beyond the past to a healthier you.

If that makes you feel uncomfortable, grab a sheet of paper, or a laptop, and construct a letter to the person who rejected you. Express everything in the letter that you found to be hurtful, or offensive. Describe in detail your pain, disappointment, feelings of frustration, and rejection. Make the letter as long as you need it to be to get your hurt out of your system. When you have completed the exercise burn the letter. This is symbolic of burning or getting rid of the hurtful emotions that have been bottled up inside of you. You may have to repeat this process several times…that is ok. The last portion of this section requires you to list as many other techniques as possible to help you deal with and release those bottled up emotions associated with your incident of rejection.

I will start you with a few, but there are many more…

Seek a professional therapist, counselor, or your ministerial official

Exercise

Write in a journal

Develop a new creative hobby such as painting, drawing, playing a musical instrument, etc. (see that creative reference to creative art here)?

Volunteer in a setting that address the type of rejection that you faced for example a domestic violence shelter, etc.

Join a twelve-step program such as Emotion Anonymous, Celebrate Recovery, etc.

Let me be clear here. Deciding to forgive is NOT the same as making the decision to restore the relationship with the person who harmed or violated you.

Forgiveness requires you to make the decision to forgive…to release the anger, bitterness, resentment, shame, etc. that is inside of you.

Reconciliation requires the decision to restore the relationship to wholeness based on the work, commitment, etc. by both parties. Take responsibility for your work.

NEVER place yourself in a situation where you will be violated, abused, or mistreated by anyone! You deserve more than abuse!

"No Extra Baggage"

I checked my baggage before my departure.
I am traveling light.

My destination is forward, I have accumulated a lot of extra
baggage during my journey, but now I am traveling light.

This train has always kept me on schedule, kept me on track.
I have paused on my journey, but the train never stopped.

At the last station, the conductor purged some of my baggage.
At first, I was stunned, angered, and shocked.
I had my ticket, my admittance, my purpose for being there!

I took inventory of my baggage, what was missing? What was
discarded?
Bitterness, anger, guilt, the need for approval of others…?
I held onto these bags for so long, I took comfort in my discomfort.

Now, I AM REALLY TRAVELING LIGHT.

What is left? How can I move forward? How can I press onward?
I don't know where I am going and traveling light is like traveling in
the dark, still looking for the light. This is strange, yet, exciting,
exhilarating!

Now I am reborn, redirected, renewed, repositioned, revitalized, and
restored. I am a shell of my former self.
I am traveling light. I am still collecting parcels for the remainder of
my journey, but my focus is not the same… my luggage is not
battered, blemished, bruised, tattered, torn or beaten. My cargo
contains instruments that charter my future course.
I am traveling light.

2   7 x 70 or something like that:
Forgiveness, the Missing Ingredient

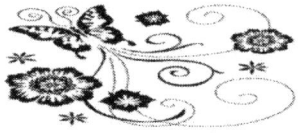

Matthew 18:21-23 Then came Peter to him, and said, Lord, how often shall my brother sin against me, and I forgive him? till seven times? Jesus saith unto him, I say not unto thee, Until seven times: but, Until seventy times seven.

Let me start out by sharing with you that forgiveness has been one of the most difficult feats for me to accomplish after learning to love myself!

I have NOT been a forgiving person. I still struggle with this at times. Because I came from a place of pain...I am not a trusting person, and I operate from a place of skepticism. Interestingly enough, when I first read that bible scripture, not only did I turn it around (7x 70 instead of 70x7, as if the total would change), but I used the scripture to allow me to keep score.

Now, I didn't just forgive, 490 times, but I began to keep score of those who offended and mistreated me.   In my mind, I would begin to forgive after 490 interactions with you. Looking back, it doesn't make a difference how I looked at the scripture, my thinking was wrong.

My heart was so weighted down with unforgiveness.

I had unforgiveness for others, but especially for myself.

This chapter is short because I am still embracing my desire to be obedient to the Word of God that He has given me to forgive instantly and have zero recall. I am a work in progress.

"Dis-Engaged Submission"

How does one fully, willfully submit when the mind is dis-engaged in the process?

The heart desires total submission, for it understands submission's greatest rewards!

My flesh has been on its own course of self-destruction since the beginning of my earthly formation...warring against the spirit, while my mind...dis-engaged!

My mind dis-engaged, dis-enfranchised, distant from submission!

Submission to God, submission from those things that I know... without thought are right!
Submission to a purpose and plan greater than my existence!

This internal struggle is raged on daily in subconscious crevices, devoid of light.

Superficially... my thoughts appear to have cognitive essence, but the deeper frequency lays dormant buried within!

Below...deep within the war rages on!

I struggle...though the battle has already been fought...the war has been won!

I stand in victory, yet I NEVER had to fight!

Freedom is right within my reach...
To submit is to gain that victory...to engage the mind, and the heart in a war against the flesh!

To willfully submit...to taste VICTORY is greater than any temporary satisfaction that can ever be reached a byproduct of the flesh! I have engaged, my mind with my spirit...I am conscious...my eyes are open, my spirit renewed!

I SUBMIT! I SUBMIT LORD!
I WILLFULLY SUBMIT!

3 Black Eye on my S.O.U.L. The Trauma of Domestic Violence...

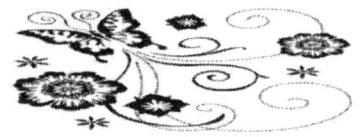

He loaded the double barrel shot gun, aimed it, and pulled the trigger. The gun clicked. He pulled the trigger again, and I heard the gun click for a second time. I was still alive...but for how much longer!? I glanced up at the ceiling and mumbled a prayer under my breath. My breathing was shallow, and my heart was racing. I absolutely refused to show fear. Not this time! Tears filled my eyes, but I refused to drop one tear.

Will was my first boyfriend. This was the man to whom I lost my virginity. I was seventeen, and he was twenty-three years old.

At first, it started off good; he was the street wise bad boy, and I was the innocent, sheltered rebellious teenager. (I thought about my innocence after writing this...although, I had given my virginity to him, my innocence was gone long before).

My two-year relationship spiraled out of control into a nightmare that I barely escaped with my life. I had been the victim of his physical abuse for two years as I suffered in silence from physical, mental, and emotional abuse. I had been slapped in public, and punched in private by Will, but this time his threats of killing me had resulted in a cocked

gun at my temple. I will never forget the cold steel pressed against my sweaty skin. He told me many times before,

"If I can't have you, then no one will."

Each time he said it, I knew in my heart I was closer to dying! I knew this was abuse, but I was in too deep and I didn't know how to get out without him killing me or my family. I was trapped!

I was terrified of him and I knew his threats of killing me were not without merit. Time seemed to stand still. Although I was paralyzed by fear, and chills ran down my spine, I silently vowed not to let him win. I couldn't scream, I couldn't run, and I refused to cry! I refused to beg him for my life, and my screams were silenced by my faith. I knew that I got myself into this mess, but only God could get me out. This time I had to stand up courageous and faithful or die.

I promised myself if I made it out alive not to ever allow myself to become a victim again. Somehow through divine intervention I was able to escape his abuse.

After the gun jammed several times, he started weeping and asking me for forgiveness. My only thought was to forgive him and get the hell out of the situation. He even tried to have sex with me. I couldn't believe it! He wanted me to have sex with him to prove that I loved him after he tried to kill me! I guess putting a loaded gun to my temple was his way of proving his love for me!

I told my mother about the abuse, and I left him alone, but he began to stalk me. He followed me back and forth to school, and work. I continued to stand my ground and stand up boldly against him every time I saw him!

What seemed like eternity was two weeks before he got the message and finally left me alone.

Ten years later, I found out that his behavior made him a victim.

He was killed as the result of an attempted robbery gone awry.

Although that experience changed my life, I found myself in another physically abusive relationship five years later. I was eight months pregnant with my first son, and a "gentleman" I had gone out with several times expressed his interest in dating exclusively. Kevin was interested in dating me, and "giving my child a name." He talked about the "honorable thing" to do, which was for us to get married. I wasn't pregnant with his child, so it looked as if he was gentlemanly. I was not impressed, and I just was not interested in getting married at that time, especially to a man that just appeared as my "knight in shining armor" to save me and my baby.

He seemed too good to be true. He was a handsome, intelligent, college student who always had women fawning over him. I was in a state of brokenness (emotionally) and I was not able to make a commitment. He wasn't a gentleman at all! In fact, he was a predator.

We went out a couple of times, and I had expressed to him that I was not interested in getting serious at that point in my life. I had so many major life changes occurring simultaneously such as "having a baby" and learning about parenthood that I was preoccupied with these overwhelming tasks.

After dinner one night, he asked to use my restroom prior to him driving home, and I allowed him to come in and use the restroom. This was a terrible mistake!

After using the restroom, we talked for a few minutes, and then when it was time for him to leave, he grabbed me and threw me against the couch. He held his hand over my mouth and took out a long switchblade knife. He whispered in my ear, "I will cut your f***ing baby out of your stomach and stab it to death right in front of you, and then I will kill you."

I started to cry; I couldn't understand why I was a victim again!

What had I done to deserve this!?

Kevin ripped my shirt off, and then he cut my bra off. The smell of his breath made me nauseated! He started to rub on my belly in a caressing manner much like many people do when they see pregnant women. I was repulsed by his touch! I gagged and started to vomit.

He asked me, "Why did you refuse my proposal? I told you that I wanted a baby and I would take care of you both!"

Honestly, I didn't know what to say! I knew that I didn't want to make him angrier. I felt so many emotions all at once...I was chilled with fear, mad as hot-as-hell's fire with rage, and dumbfounded. He snatched off my pants and cut off my underwear. I really got scared!!! My son kicked inside like he was defending his mother. My tears had no effect on him. I didn't know if I should passively lay still or aggressively fight. My apartment was tiny and usually I could hear my neighbors, but this time all I heard was his heavy breathing and my heart beating fast! Kevin started choking me until I just about passed out. He let me breathe and then he started biting me in my face. He bit me several times as if he wanted to take a piece of flesh with each bite. I cried, I kicked, I fought back. He took the knife out again and pressed the blade into my belly! My baby was kicking like crazy...he was fighting for his life too!

Blood started to ooze from the superficial cut.

He said, "Tanya, don't make me kill your baby."

I stopped fighting and then...he penetrated me with his penis.

His thrust inside of me seemed to go on forever! I don't know when I stopped crying, but I know that I left my body on that floor and went to a place where he could not hurt me.

Once he finished...he left quietly...just like nothing happened.

That sick bastard left his filthy, evil semen inside of me. I laid on the floor in my living room and cried out in agony and pain! I was livid! I cried all night! I think my baby cried all night too!

The next morning, I woke up, showered, and convinced myself that the best thing to do was to make a police report. I looked at my face in the mirror, my face was puffy and swollen, and I had three sets of teeth prints on my cheeks. I am a deep brown complexion, but the red fingerprint marks were clearly visible on my neck.

The police took me to a private room and took my information, as well as took pictures of my face and neck. I refused to have a rape examination because I didn't want to undergo additional trauma to my vaginal area or to my baby.

Growing up, I was the victim of molestation, now a brutal date rape. One thing I knew for sure…men could not be trusted! That truth had been proven and established too many times.

Fast forward to my late thirties and many relationships later, I began to change my mind-set about male-female relationships. I really wanted a committed loving relationship, but I didn't know how to identify the right type of men, and those men that were good to me were the men that I was least attracted to.

Like the needle in the vein of a heroin addict, I needed that closeness, the physical contact, and the intimacy. I just wanted to be loved and accepted, but I was consumed with satisfying my need for love through sex. I thought I was addicted to sex, but I was really starved for love.

During my sexual escapades, I would cry out real tears. My sexual partners thought my tears were enjoyment, but I was crying out to God for help. I was caught up; I couldn't stop having sex, even though I believed in my heart that it was wrong to have sex outside of marriage.

Each time I had sex, it provided less fulfillment, but my desires for more sex increased. With every sexual encounter, and every failed relationship, I was separating myself from God. I was searching for something that I would never find by changing sexual partners...I was searching for LOVE.

I thought the best way to address my addiction for sex was to get married, so I got married. I could satisfy my sexual desires within my marriage, and that would make everything perfect...so I thought!

Sexually, I was in a great space...I was fulfilled, but everything else was bad! I was a terrible wife! My husband never physically, emotionally, or verbally abused me. My first husband had his issues, but I was so broken that I couldn't nurture and help him heal. I heaped hurt on top of his hurt, and pain on top of his pain. We were two damaged people who married and had a damaged marriage.

Now, I had graduated from physical abuse to emotional abuse. I would no longer tolerate physical black eyes, but I had so many black eyes on my soul.

After my first and second divorce, I was finished with allowing men to hurt me! I had been hurt, and it was time to return the favor! I was an emotional disaster, but I was hiding the pain in numbness and unforgiveness. My mission was revenge.

My rules were simple:

Rule # 1: Stay in emotional control; separate sex from love.

Rule # 2: Never fall in LOVE.

Rule # 3: Refer to rules #1 and #2.

My mantra: Get them before they get you!

Man #1 was a player and he taught me the "game." He was a smooth talker, smooth dresser, and smooth lover. It was fun with him; we both understood that we were both temporary. We both knew that nothing would develop from the relationship.

Man #2 was the man that I fell in love with quickly! I violated all my own rules and I got hurt! This brother was tall, dark, handsome, and he had a perfect athletic built. He slew me with his charisma like David slew Goliath! One shot and I fell hard!

I was hooked again-and this time I was strung out!

There was just one problem…he didn't want me.

He was so smooth that the words from his lips dripped of honey…he told lies that were believable just because he told them. That man used me, well…I allowed myself to be used because I knew better, but it felt so good being with him even though we were never or rarely seen in public together. I had DE-VALUED myself…I didn't expect anything from him, and he didn't give me anything. I had a very serious soul-tie to this man, and he didn't care for me at all.

In fact, one time he was lying in bed with me, we had just finished having sex. We were having "after-glow" discussion. I am not sure how the subject changed but he started talking with me about a woman that he was interested in dating and how she rejected him. He started to weep, and I held him in my arms and cried with him. He was crying over her, and I was crying that I was a damn fool for him!

I really was a love starved damn fool!

That was the last straw! I couldn't take the hurt, the lies, the deceit, and the rejection anymore!

My relationships with men were so bad I honestly couldn't trust God. I felt as if God is male, and he made men, and men have always hurt me in some form or fashion…how could God be any different!?

I knew what I was carrying inside of me was killing me…the pain, the bitterness, the distrust, the fragmented relationships! All of it was literally killing me. I wanted to so desperately to be loved. I started with God. I asked him to forgive me for searching around in the darkness for love, although I thought it was just in the darkness of bedrooms and under the covers; it was much deeper than that. The anger I had towards God began to melt away.

I began to trust God, and then I took a major step and finally forgave my father. I wrote a letter to him and addressed it to the last known address. I sent two copies; one was certified mail, and the other regular mail. Only one letter came back. I am not sure if he ever got the other letter, but I forgave him for his absence, and for not providing and protecting me from child predators and molestation. I also forgave him for not teaching me about male-female relationships. Most of all I forgave him for not loving me. This was a two-year process of forgiveness.

God birthed newness in my womb. I experienced a cleansing from the souls of the men of my past, and a cleansing of the yearnings of my addiction to both sex and the longing to be loved through the act of sex.

The layers of pain were slowly stripped away, and those black eyes on my soul were healed.

In 2008, God gave me some words to meditate on to facilitate my healing. These words are: REjuvenate, REstore, REnew, REcharge, REcreate, REfocus, REalign, REvive, REflect, REconnect, REjoice, REvitalize, REposition, REdeemed.

In 2009, I met a wonderful man that God placed in my life to love me.

On the first date he said, "I am here as the result of your prayers and I promise to never lie to you, to never cheat on you, and to never hurt you."

There were certain things that he said that I knew in my spirit, he was the one! I knew it and he knew it on the first date. It wasn't love at first sight; there were no lightning bolts and fireworks…there was a quiet gentle confirmation that he was the one in my spirit. We were married in 2011 and have been together since.

RElate

In this chapter, I shared many examples of verbal, physical, mental, emotional, and sexual abuse. Unfortunately for me, there were several others not listed. It took intense therapy and self-help materials to understand that I was worthy to be protected, treated with love and respect, and free from violence of any kind.

As a matter of fact, the title, Black Eye On My S.O.U.L. refers to the emotional violence suffered while Seeking Out Unhealthy Love, and how those scars healed much slower. My point here is that although your experience may not have resulted in physical abuse, abuse is abuse.

How can you relate to the experiences of physical, mental, emotional, verbal, sexual abuse? Write your experiences below.

Some people believe physical violence is the worse form of domestic abuse, but physical scars are not the only type of *scars*. What type of emotional, verbal, sexual, or mental abuse have left lasting scars in your life?

R<u>E cover</u>

It is important to begin to understand why you feel the way that you do in order to allow yourself to continue to be a victim of any kind of abuse or violence. No matter the form of abuse…you DO NOT have to remain a victim. One decision to change your life can make you a victor instead of a victim. Recovery from abuse often takes assistance from professionals. Therapist, counselors, or other mental health professionals can all be instrumental in assisting you in the recovery process.

It is natural and normal to feel afraid…I have been there! A loaded shotgun placed at my head was scary! There was another time I had a knife placed at my belly while I was pregnant…that is scary! I didn't do anything to deserve this abuse, but I had to learn to value myself. I am not disillusioned. I made it out safe but not unscathed. Many victims of violence never make it out.

If you are in an abusive relationship currently, GET HELP!

You may have to get assistance from a domestic violence shelter, develop a safety plan, get help from a trusted friend or relative, get a personal protection order from your local courthouse, etc.

Write down your feelings about the incident, and the person who hurt you.

_____

_____

_____

_____

_____

_____

_____

_____

_____

_____

_____

_____

_____

_____

What were some of the signs of abuse that were there? How did you ignore them, or were you not knowledgeable of the signs?

_____

_____

_____

_____

_____

_____

_____

_____

_____

_____

_____

_____

_____

_____

_____

_____

_____

_____

_____

RElease

One of the greatest forms of releasing the pain of the past is by becoming knowledgeable.

Here are some resources:

The National Domestic Violence Hotline: 1-800-799-SAFE (7233)

https://www.thehotline.org

www.emotionalanonymous.org

1-651-647-9712

Emotions Anonymous is an international fellowship of men and women who desire to improve their emotional well-being. EA members come together in weekly meetings for the purpose of working toward recovery from any sort of emotional difficulties. EA members are of diverse ages, races, economic status, social and educational backgrounds. The only requirement for membership is a desire to become well emotionally

"Black Eye on my S.O.U.L."

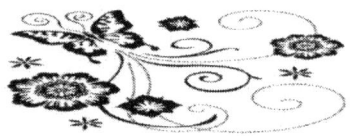

The words "I'm sorry" does not erase the black eye that you left on my soul. Each time you get angry, you yell, you rant, and you rave…

You cause another black eye on my soul.

Yes, you say, "I'm sorry," and yes, you apologize. Yes, you say, "It will never happen again." You even go as far as saying, "I meant it when I said it, but that's not how I really feel."

I'm sorry doesn't erase the black eye you left on my soul.

Out of the abundance of the heart the mouth speaks, is there so much pain deep in your soul that your words lash out at me?

Opposites attract they say, but it seems your brokenness attracted my brokenness. Years of emotional, verbal, physical and sexual abuse once jilted my soul.

I removed myself, healed myself and willed myself to rise from pain.

I am a graduate- I won't; I refuse to allow anyone to abuse me. I will fight back or die fighting!

There will never be another black eye on my soul.

"Broken Heart-I-tis"

Psalm 2008

Oh, merciful Father I cry out to thee.

Lift my head.

Dry my tears.

Heal my heart, Lord.

How long must I nurse this wounded heart?

Give me a fleshy heart in place of this stony heart

Love me like days of old long before my adornment with humanly clothes.

Heal me of this "Dis-ease" called broken heart-I-tis.

Restore

Renew

Refresh my soul.

Amen.

4   Daddy, When Are You Coming Back?

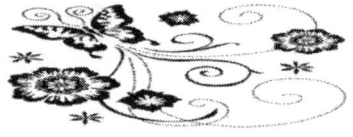

He picked me up, hugged, kissed me, and said, "Baby, I love you. I'll be back."

Although, I could not articulate my feelings at that time, I knew something wasn't quite right. It was a sad time for me, and I didn't understand why he had to leave me.

"Daddy when are you coming back?"

"Soon honey," he reassured me.

That was more than forty years ago. I have not seen him since.

His absence left a hole in my soul that took me many years to understand. Only God could fill the void, but before learning this, I attempted to fill the void with drugs, sex, food, and the desire to please people as the remedies to relieve the pain I was experiencing.

I can recall prior to the age of twelve someone called me a bastard child. I specifically remember the hurt and humiliation I felt, but the curiosity of defining the term bastard was equally important, so I rushed home to look the word "Bastard" up in the dictionary. This is what I found:

1. an illegitimate child (not recognized as lawful offspring, born of parents not married to each other; not rightly deduced or inferred: illogical, departing from the regular); illegal, not authorized for good usage.
2. something that is spurious (see SPURIOUS 3a), irregular, inferior, or of questionable origin
3. an offensive or disagreeable person
All I did was to be born!

From that day forward I carried that rejection around with me… and when I discovered these words in the Bible, I knew I wasn't alone. Jeremiah 20:14 described my feelings exactly:

14 Cursed be the day wherein I was born: let not the day wherein my mother bare me be blessed.

15 Cursed be the man who brought tidings to my father, saying, A man child is born unto thee; making him very glad.

16 And let that man be as the cities which the LORD overthrew, and repented not: and let him hear the cry in the morning, and the shouting at noontide;

17 Because he slew me not from the womb; or that my mother might have been my grave, and her womb to be always great with me.

18 Wherefore came I forth out of the womb to see labor and sorrow, that my days should be consumed with shame?

Job 10:19 I should have been as though I had not been; I should have been carried from the womb to the grave.

There is no father's name listed on my birth certificate, there was no daddy to cover, protect, or love me… My mom loved me, but I always felt there was something missing…the fact that I haven't seen or heard from my father in more than 45 years added to the pain of the rejection.

Abandoned, cast aside…yep, that was me! The "R" in my middle name was for Rejection!

The first sixteen years of my life, I was angry, but I couldn't identify the source of anger. I knew something was missing in my family of origin, but in all honesty, there were so many other families in my neighborhood in the same predicament absent fathers was common. In fact, the first time I had seen a father in a home, outside of television shows, was at a sleep over in high school. I can distinctly remember asking my best friend Carolyn, *"Does your father live here?"* She said, *"Yes."*

I was dumbfounded. I asked, *"Does he sleep here every night?"*

She indicated, *"Tanya, my dad has lived here all my life."*

That weekend was one of my best weekends living in a home with a dad, even if he wasn't my father. Seeing my friends with their fathers caused me to become sensitive to the absence of my father. The anger I felt grew into rage, rebellion, and blatant disrespect for my mother.

I saw too many adult situations, and I was exposed to too many instances of my mother's boyfriends molesting me or making inappropriate comments towards me. Although my mother was the responsible person there taking care of me to the best of her ability, my hostility was directed towards her, and my longing was for my father. I made lots of excuses for his absence, and in my mind, he was the hero, and she was the villain. I remember vividly making up stories each summer about going away with my real family for the summer…only just like my biological father never came back for me neither did my make-believe family. I was sad or angry all the time…but I couldn't reach out to ask for help.

I can recall hearing the term, *dysfunctional* used as a reference to people associated with broken homes. Now, there was a term that defined me... I was dysfunctional.

I didn't know my home was broken, and I didn't know how to fix it! I was always a reader, and I read material that was on a higher level of my comprehension. I remember reading the popular magazine, Psychology Today, articles by the Psychologist Dr. Joyce Brothers, and books by Norman Vincent Peale. "The Power of a Positive Mind," and "I'm Ok, You're Ok" were the books that changed the trajectory of my future at thirteen years old. I read so many self-help books that related to building self-esteem, self-confidence, and self-respect. I had no idea that that is a form of therapy called bibliotherapy.

Although, I had to read the books with the aid of a dictionary, and the encyclopedia, I began to understand that my plight of being born a bastard, dysfunctional, black girl did not have to define me my entire life. These terms were descriptive words that I could refuse to use to define me.

RElate

How are you able to relate to that story? Did people negatively impact your self-esteem by name calling or shaming you? Did you grow up without a parent? How did that absent parent impact your life?

_____

_____

_____

_____

_____

_____

_____

_____

_____

REcover

A huge part of recovery is dealing with the past, but for years I refused to acknowledge those hurtful feelings. I covered up my pain and denied that those hurtful events occurred. Refusing to acknowledge the pain is also refusing to heal. What experience from your past hurt you, and left you numb, in denial, or grieving? There is so much healing power in the writing process. Try this exercise. Write a letter to the person who hurt you. Don't mail the letter, just release the pain.

RElease

Now place the letter in an envelope, seal it, and mail it...no return address. The letter cannot come back...no need to address it to the person who harmed you either. Place the pain in the envelope and release it.

"Who is the Father to the Fatherless?

Psalms 68:5   A father of the fatherless, and a judge of the widows, is God in his holy habitation.

Romans 8:14
For as many as are led by the Spirit of God, they are the sons of God. 15 For ye have not received the spirit of bondage again to fear; but ye have received the Spirit of adoption, whereby we cry, Abba, Father. 16 The Spirit itself beareth witness with our spirit, that we are the children of God:

I was adopted by my Heavenly Father, and I am no longer a bastard child or an orphan!

5 Vaginal Sinkhole...Under the Covers with Sin, NO MORE!

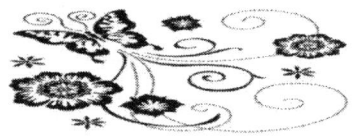

For many years I struggled with addiction. My struggle raged on even before I was conscious that I was engaged in a struggle. This was a Battle for my SOUL!

My addiction and drug of choice...SEX!

I was not addicted to sex like many sex addicts who become compulsive in behavior that is offensive or abusive to others. Nor did I have to have sex with anyone, anytime, or anywhere. I didn't get involved in pornography, excessive masturbation, or become a sexual offender of any kind. My sexual addiction harmed me, and that still resulted in sexual sin. All sin leads to death...spiritual death, and before long, an accelerated physical death. The enemy really had me deceived into believing that I was "better" because l was in a "quasi-committed" relationship-only one partner at a time. I was always justifying my behavior. I was caught up into thinking I was not really a sinner. I know now all that is foolishness! Lies that I told myself and lies that I believed about myself.

I was addicted in every sense of the word. l wanted sex every day, and I could not get enough of it.

I am embarrassed by my behavior looking back now.

Like a needle in the vein of a heroin addict, I needed that closeness, the physical contact...that intimacy. I didn't feel whole or complete until I was in the arms of a lover.

So why the title, Vaginal Sinkhole?

Well, a sink hole or swallow hole occurs when there is a depression in the ground caused by some form of collapse of the surface layers. Sink holes have been used for centuries in ancient civilizations as disposal sites for various types of waste materials. (google.com)

A vagina is a canal in a female mammal that leads from the uterus to the external orifice of the genital canal (websterdictionary.com)

My vagina, a mysterious unrelated body part hidden away, "down there." It had a single purpose in my adolescent mind, but the two terms collided in my life when I was molested at the age of eleven.

My innocence was lost, and the seed of fornication was sown into my heart. Maybe sown into my vagina is a more accurate description.

It was at this time when I began to understand that some men would go to great extremes to have sex, even if it was predatory with minor children.

I began to understand that the rejection that I constantly endured had exceptions.

I was desirable after all, even if it was at night, hidden, or converted like a secret undercover spy mission. The details were to be kept "TOP SECRET."

No one asked/no one told. It was a dirty little secret; best unspoken, taboo, and unconscionable. A friend of the family wanted to fondle my breast, and I wanted the money that he offered me. It later turned out to be a bad decision. To think back about me making a decision like that frightens me. My future could have turned out so different!

God's grace and mercy covered me.

There was a song made famous in 1979, written and performed by singer and recording artist Donna Summer entitled, "Bad Girl." The lyrics described a young girl as a prostitute. The song had the perfect beat and lyrics that described the trajectory of my future life as a prostitute. It was one of my favorite songs. I was the dirty, nasty bad girl, or so I thought about myself at the age of eleven when the song debuted. I vividly recall singing, chanting, and feeding my psyche with the words of that song.

Fast forward several years, I began being sexually active. I gave my virginity away at the age of sixteen to a man, twenty-five years old. I was not mature enough to make that type of decision. No one taught or encouraged me to wait until marriage to have sex. I was taught to make the decision when I felt I was ready to start having sex. I was always an avid reader, so I was well educated about my sexual reproductive organs, my choices for birth control, and how to protect myself from sexually transmitted diseases. All the books prepared me for those type of adult decisions. I lacked wisdom to understand the emotional, mental, and spiritual consequences associated with having sex outside of marriage. In fact, I remember when I started my menstrual cycle at twelve, I remember the books written congratulated me on becoming a "Woman."

There was just one small problem, I took that literally! There was ONLY one WOMAN in my mother's house, and it wasn't me. So, when I started having sex, I let my mother know she could no longer tell me what to do because, I was a woman. I had rationalized several factors into this STUPID equation.

First, my mother gave birth to me at the age of sixteen, so I was already ahead of her decision-making process. Second, I knew about birth control, and sexual transmitted diseases, etc. Hell! at that point, I was having orgasms. The literature I read indicated, most women didn't have multiple organisms, so I was an exception. These were excellent reasons to confront my mother! However, I failed to evaluate several other factors before electing to confront my mother.

First, I had no job, no money, no place to go, and no education. I didn't bring anything of significant value or worth into the household. Last of all, and most importantly, I was disrespecting my mother. My mother rendered the most profuse behind whipping I had ever had at that point in my life! The firework of stars, stripes, and rockets that I thought I experienced during my first orgasm failed in comparison to those delivered at the hands of my mother!

Whatever lying, demonic spirit that whispered in my ear to encourage me to rise up with a false sense of pride and a super inflated ego hid its ugly head when my mother beat that courage out of me.

All the books I read didn't prepare me for what I would experience.

It's funny, it has been more than thirty years since the incident and my legs tremble, my heart is racing, and my breathing is faster. The lesson I learned was to NEVER attempt to rise up full strength at my mother. I did try several other occasions, but I never did it at full strength.

Sex was good, but I was consumed with sex, and yet I am Christian. I attend a church where the Word of God is taught! I know scriptures that talk about fornicators having their place in the pit of hell, yet I was divided between my love for God and my love and need for sex.

In reality, it was my need for love and acceptance that fueled my desire for sex. It would take me many years to discover this truth.

I was so strung out at my "rock bottom" that I would cry out to God in the midst of my sexual encounter. Those tears were real tears, screams of agony and gut-wrenching pain from the depth of my being, but they were masked to appear that the man I was sexually active with was sexually satisfying me!

My screams of passion were really screams to the Father-whom I knew was looking down on me in my filth! As the tears flowed my heart would break, knowing that once again I had chosen my fleshly desires over pleasing God. Each time I had sex, it provided less and less fulfillment. My desires for more sex increased, and my fulfillment decreased.

With every sexual encounter, and every failed relationship, I was separating myself from God and searching for something that I would never find by changing sexual partners...LOVE.

This cycle began to spin out of control! I was decaying from the inside out.

My relatively stable layer of self-worth was caving in under the weight of the guilt and shame as the vaginal sinkhole hole began to consume more of my essence with each sexual encounter.

I grew up in Detroit, Michigan, and my mother raised me and my siblings as a single mother. It is very important to share my story, and my story alone, but can I really separate my upbringing from that of my parents?

The fabric of my life is from the woven threads of my parents. The sins of my parents were passed onto me...generational curses, and I have repeated some of those things, that is until I learned of the Power of the Holy Spirit to bind and break those demonic curses.

As a young child, my mother displayed open affection, and expressed love to us, but there was always something missing. Years later I understood that the balance was off kilter because there was no father figure in the home. The absence of my father as the provider, protector, and example of healthy relationships had affected me more than I was willing to believe or admit. In fact, it played a major contribution to the correlation of both my sexual promiscuousness, and my attraction to unhealthy relationships.

Several years ago, my grandmother and I were talking, and she told me, "Baby, promiscuousness is any sex outside of marriage."

Of course, I took her words of wisdom outside the context of our conversation and I was furious. I thought my granny was calling me promiscuous. I was in fact, unmarried and having sex. It didn't matter if I had one sexual partner or many, I was still promiscuous and still in SIN! My shame and guilt were calling me out, those things that I did in the dark under the covers were really coming into the light. My magic formula for hiding my addiction-my magic cure to having more sex-MARRIAGE! So, I got married. I thought marriage would solve all my problems. It would fill in the gaps. I would become whole, and complete. I was so deceived! In marriage, I had all the legal, legitimate sex-but something was still missing! I was missing LOVE!

In my first marriage, I didn't know that two emotionally damaged individuals do NOT equal a healthy, loving, Godly marriage. We both loved each other, but we did not know how to love each other in a Godly manner. I was so broken; the infrastructure of my heart was badly in need of Godly transformation. The hurt in my life was transferred and magnified in his life. He tried to love me as best he could, but the surmounting pain heaped on top of pain resulted in our demise.

I vowed to never marry again, but I desired to have sex within the parameters of marriage. I married a second time, but this time I thought it would be for the remainder of my life. The first warning sign of this marriage looming failure was my justification of our spiritual incompatibility. I am not blaming anyone. I married two good men, but I was not good for them and they were not God's best for me. In both marriages, the common denominator was me.

I know that both marriages failed because I was still seeking LOVE from human beings rather than learning to love God and allowing God to heal me from my past hurt. I needed to heal from the void caused by the absence of my father, where the distrust of men and the spirit of rejection were rooted.

I was still looking for LOVE and acceptance.

My second divorce devastated me! I was devastated because I worked hard to change my past behavior. I married a man totally opposite of my first marriage-in every perspective. I had superficially done things different, but I still did not address the real problem-ME! There was a lot more internal damage than I initially thought. I was an emotional disaster!

The emotional devastation was equal to that of hurricane Hugo, Wanda, and Katrina. I hid it well, or so I thought! I was simply masking the pain in numbness with unforgiveness at its root. My weight had ballooned to 300 pounds, rather than using sex as my comfort, I had replaced it with food. I decided that I had been hurt enough, and it was time to return the favor! Little did I know I would become my next VICTIM! The greatest amount of pain would be inflicted on ME!

My first recourse-SEX-with a vengeance!

I was going after the men who hurt me…my mission was different.

Rule #1: Stay in emotional control: separate sex from love.

Rule #2: Never fall in LOVE.

Rule #3: Refer to rules #1 and #2!

My new mantra: Get them before they get you!

Man, number one was a "real player." He taught me how to perfect my craft, and how to play the game from a "real players" point of view. He made getting into sin fun, even enticing…and I was perfecting my craft, learning from an old pro. He had been playing for much longer than I had, and he was much better at playing the game than I ever could become. I just lost steam, and the game got old! That should have been an indication right then that I could not "play the game!"

Man, number two…he fell in love quickly, and I was out of the relationship quick! He was a casualty of the game, and I left him by the wayside holding his heart. He loved me unconditionally, and that was not enough! The seeds of heartache and destruction were sown for the harvest of pain that I would soon reap.

Man, number three…I fell in love quickly, and I got hurt. This was a good set up by the enemy. He was tall, dark, handsome, and he oozed charisma. He slayed me, like David slayed Goliath! I was smitten.

One shot and I fell hard! I was hooked, an addict again! Strung out! I wanted him with every ounce of my being. I wanted to do more than secretly meet in hotel rooms and have sex. I wanted him to make a commitment to me, and for us to have that special connection. There was just one problem. He did not want me!

How could I be so foolish to think that the game would end any other way!?

I was NEVER going to win! I was a fool. The players changed, but the game was the same.

The payment for SIN IS ALWAYS DEATH!

I learned quickly that sin will make you bend all the rules. It will make you compromise all your morals, all your values, and sin will make you lie. I lied to others, and I lied to myself.

Things that I said, "I will NEVER DO," I did!

I had de-VALUED myself and sunk to a new low. I was ashamed to be in the presence of my family and friends. I stood in constant shame and guilt before God. The veil of rejection that I wore now had the added adornments of shame and guilt. I did those things in SIN, in search for LOVE.

Thank God for his MERCY because if it had not been for Christ, I would be on a fast track to the pit of hell! Passing go and collecting two hundred dollars would not be an option! The game that I was playing could have cost me my soul, lost in hell's eternal fire. Thank God for his word! Thank God for the cleansing and restoration that occurs when we allow the Word of God to radiate and penetrate our hearts and minds!

I began to listen to the Holy Spirit inside of me. I let the Spirit of God minister to my heart and deliver me.

First, I sought forgiveness from God, and then when I was able, I forgave myself. I forgave my earthly father for his absence, and then I forgave my mother for her choices. I learned that in order to be forgiven, I must forgive. Forgiving requires the absence of blame!

Forgiveness is the missing piece to acceptance of God's LOVE! That is the purpose of John 3:16.

I had no idea of how devastating the consequences of my sin would be. I have been a victim of date rape at knifepoint, and a victim of mental, physical, and emotional abuse. The word of God indicates that the wages of sin is death. I practiced deliberate sexual sin, but not without a high price.

Thank God that it did not cost me my life! God, in his loving mercy, snatched me from the grips of bondage and hell! I thank God for these experiences. Although, I am not proud of this part of my life, I am not ashamed anymore either. God birthed newness in my womb; I experienced a cleansing from the souls of the men of my past, and a cleansing of the yearnings of my addiction.

The layers of pain have slowly been stripped away from my soul, and I am walking in the REstoration of Christ...Free from Sexual Addiction!

I must share my story; it allows me to stay accountable and out of hiding in those darkened rooms, under the covers with Tom, Dick, Harry, and?

No amount of sex was ever going to fulfill the love of Jesus Christ. No man can ever fill the void that a life without the loving personal relationship with the Creator provides. That vaginal sink hole in my life was synonymous to my gaping hole in my whole spirit.

In 2008, God gave me some words to meditate to facilitate my healing. They are as follows: REjuvenate, REstore, REnew, REcharge, REcreate, REfocus, REalign, REvive, REflect, REconnect, REjoice, REvitalize, REposition, and REdeemed!

Now I understand why I never desired to use my middle name, which begins with the letter "R," but now my middle name is all of those "RE words." I laugh now because it is more than a REbuilding, or REbranding. It is a REBIRTH, a RENEWAL, and a RECONNECTION to the Father.

It took many years before I could talk about the vaginal sink hole, the shame, and guilt became unbearable.

Thank God; that was then, this is NOW!

"I am Gonna Make me a Man"

I couldn't wait on God to provide for me what I could provide for myself, only I didn't know what He knew.

I decided God is too slow, too busy, or He just needs some help, so "I am going to make me a man." I took matters into my own hands.

I started out being the provider, the protector, and the lead. I had the car. I had the home. I had the income.

Everything I had, I worked for. All that was missing was my man.

Now it was time to place the man on the scene. Yes, I thought I could place the man in my life like God placed Adam in the Garden of Eden. I started out by piecing together the "Perfect Dysfunctional Man-Made Man."

It took many years later to learn that his dysfunctions were my dysfunctions and those I didn't like in him, I hated in me.

I enabled him, and I was co-dependent to my own addictions.

He didn't work; he didn't have to. I had a job. After all, I stepped up my role as the provider. I worked two and sometimes three jobs to supply our needs.

I led him, fed him, provided for him, and protected him. Every role that is associated with the male dominant in our society, I provided to him.

His every need was provided for by me. I had it covered. This included his cigarettes, his alcohol, and his street mood altering drugs.

Just like the Father took care of Adam, I took care of my "Perfectly Dysfunctional woMan-Made Man."

He wasn't educated; he didn't have to be…I was. No diploma or GED required. He was streetwise and that was all that was necessary. I took care of him!

He validated me, sexed me, and when he was there, he fed my desire for a man. A piece of a man, a broken man…that was all I desired. I couldn't ask for more, I wasn't capable of giving more. I didn't believe that I deserved more.

6 V2127690A; Welfare, Food Stamps, and the Poverty Mentality

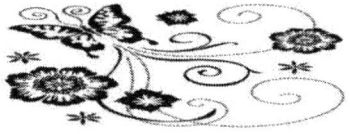

V2127690A was my welfare case number for ten years.

At the age of eighteen, I got pregnant with my first child. I never gave birth to that child, but I gave birth to a cycle of welfare dependence that lasted for ten years. In fact, it has been more than twenty-five years since I have been off welfare, and yet that prison number still easily rolls off my tongue. I can quote it as easily as my social security number, driver's license, and my birthdate.

I learned for me that welfare dependency was permeated in my psyche long after my ten-year poverty stint ended. This poverty mentality was deeply entrenched far down into my inner core.

The poverty line is defined as the smallest amount of money a person or a family needs to live on or buy what is needed. People who are below this line are classified as poor. This line is used to decide who can get extra help with things like food, shelter or medical care.

Growing up, I vividly recall messages of lack fictionalized on television, and portrayed in my daily reality. As a matter of fact, I thought all African American people were poor, and all Caucasian people were rich based on television, and my daily reality growing up in my community. I assumed that everyone struggled like we struggled.

My mother struggled to provide for her four children, working double shifts as a cleaning woman. She didn't receive child support, so there was always an abundance of lack.

Things that are considered basic necessities in this country, such as toothpaste, deodorant, soap, paper towel, napkins, mouthwash, and dental floss, just to name a few items were normally scarce. I recall brushing my teeth with baking soda, dishwashing liquid, and soap. I used baking soda as deodorant, and often washed my hair, and clothing with dish washing liquid.

Name brand items were luxury items, and government subsidized food items such as cheese, dried milk, canned meats, and canned juices were typical staples. The embarrassment associated with utilizing paper food stamps to pay for groceries was a common occurrence for me growing up in the 1970s. I cringed every time my mother sent me to the store with a list and food stamps.

At the time, I wasn't mature enough to be grateful for the food, the utilities, clothing, and a roof over my head. Instead, as an immature child, my focus was on everything that either I couldn't have or didn't have.

Fast forward to my young adult years. I gave birth to my first son, and the cycle of welfare dependency generation: TWO.

The struggle of making ends meet, more days of the month on the calendar than money to provide for my children became my reality. Oh, then there was the additional factor there was no financial support from my sons' fathers.

The Poverty cycle had been REPEATED.

There were many factors to take into consideration, poor planning, ignorance, or a subliminal message from my past. The lack, struggle, guilt, and shame were all my reality.

One constant principle my mother instilled in me was that NO ONE owes me anything! Even though we needed government assistance to supplement our deficiencies, I was reminded often to work hard to take care of myself, and to take pride in working. My mother never raised me to think I was entitled to anyone providing for me.

Today, according to federal guidelines that define poverty, I am no longer poor. There are times when I catch myself not practicing delayed gratification, or spending money on things I see rather than budgeting. Impulse purchases are still a struggle.

Learning to become a producer of services and goods is my focus these days. Trillions of dollars are spent in the global economy every day. I can make a conscience decision to invest in property, stocks, bonds, mutual funds, and other investments that will help my money to grow. I have a choice to continue the poverty legacy or pass on a legacy to my children, and grandchildren with abundance and multiple streams of income.

RElate

Poverty is more than lack of money. Poverty has a smell, a stench of its own. Poverty is gloomy, dingy, and dirty. Poverty will cause people to act in primal ways to fulfill normal drives for food, clothing, shelter, etc. A person who has never been poor cannot understand it, and a person who has been poor has to fight to combat it!

How can you relate to poverty? How can you relate to not having enough of the basic necessities such as food, shelter, clothing, etc?

What long term effects has poverty had in your life?

Do you believe that people who are poor are lazy, or that it is their fault that they are poor? What brought about the shift in your thinking? What has been a catalyst for change?

_____

_____

_____

_____

_____

_____

_____

_____

_____

_____

RE cover

If you have been poor, how did you change your financial status?

_____

_____

_____

What suggestions would you offer someone else struggling with a poverty mentality?

R E lease

The biggest part of change is recognizing the need for change. Once we recognize the need for change then making steps to change becomes necessary. In this illustration learning to budget money, journaling your spending habits, and understanding how to empower yourself are examples of ways to become released from the grip of a poverty mentality. Education is vital to changing behavior.

What can you do to change your circumstances and free yourself of an impoverished mentality?

7   The Throw Away Woman Syndrome & The Throw Away Wife Syndrome   *"TAWS"*

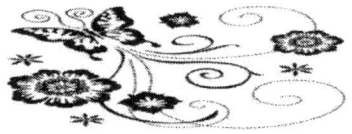

"I don't ever want to get married. I just want to have my babies and not be bothered with a husband. Men are nothing but a lot of trouble."

"Men cannot be trusted. They all cheat, they all lie, they are not any good."

"A good man is hard to find."

"They are all going to lie to you."

These are all messages that I heard growing up. They were not from one specific person, but more from a combination of my experiences. I had witnessed my mother involved in a series of toxic relationships that left her broken. As a child, I didn't know all the details, but I pieced together enough of her pain to understand that I wanted no parts of dealing with men of this caliber. Ironically, I didn't see a different type of man regularly in real life to base my choices for future mates.

I believed the only kind of man for me was the knight in shining armor that would ride up on his magical horse, plant a long, loving kiss on my lips, and whisk me away to a beautiful kingdom where we would live happily ever after. Every fairy tale ended just like that. I read a

lot, and the story was always the same. Why would my story end any different?

There was just one problem. My story didn't start off like the fairy tales. I wasn't Rapunzel with the magical hair. My hair was curly kinky. I wasn't born in a castle in a kingdom far far away, and there were no seven dwarfs, evil stepmother, fairy godmother, or magical mirror. Fairy tales were cool if they were true, but then they would not have the same fascination and appeal, would they?

Unless we as human beings make a conscientious effort to break out of cultural paradigms, we are prone to repeat behavior from our past. This occurs whether we are aware of the paradigms or not.

Indeed, I am challenged by the concept of repeating my past now that is no fairy tale this is reality.

My point?

Those same types of men that I disliked, despised, and thought to be deviant, dysfunctional, and downright the "bottom of the barrel" turned out to be the bad boys that I was attracted to…in the beginning.

Absent a real life, flesh and blood example of the ideal man, a street savvy, bad boy, abusive, irresponsible man became the next best candidate for my future suitor.

I began dating at the age of sixteen and gave away my virginity at seventeen.

In the beginning, Will protected me. He was a predator and understood it was important to learn my vulnerabilities before exposing his true intentions. As his intended victim I walked into his web of deception with my eyes wide shut, without the knowledge of the web that I had become entangled in until the trap was set in plain sight.

By the time the trap sprung in place, only God could help me get out of the hell hole because my grave would have been my final destination. Ironically, my thoughts about men in general became my self-fulfilling reality. Relationship after relationship was filled with fresh opportunities of the same dysfunctionalism. It is as my life was broken on the repeat cycle, or my forehead flashed with bright neon lights that screamed to my future abuser *"hurt me"*, *"mistreat me"* *"abuse me"*.

The good guys I dated seemed boring, nerdy, or there was some other insignificant reason for my lack of interest. I can think of at least three men from my past that would have made excellent husbands. In fact, at my last check, each one has celebrated long term marriages of twenty or more years. I trust and believe God my life unfolded the way it was supposed to unfold. They were good men, but mentally and emotionally I could not sustain a healthy relationship.

I gave birth to my first son at the age of twenty, and my second son at the age of twenty-three. Both of my children were born out of wedlock, and both had different fathers.

REPEAT.

REWIND...the cycle of dysfunction in my life was now on steroids.

I carried so much guilt and shame in my life because of my religious beliefs of premarital sex being forbidden, yet I was fully engaged in premarital sex. As a matter of fact, I was having lots of sex...only now I was pregnant, and my secret was no longer concealed.

My belief system was so messed up that I saw little value in myself, and sex was the equivalent to love.

I thought a good remedy for the poor decisions in my life was to rectify the guilt and shame by getting married.

The bible indicates that it is better to marry rather than burn with passion...right? Marriage was the only corrective course of action to take to make my life complete.

We married on my birthday, January 20, 1994.

I had cried, manipulated, and cajoled him for eight years, until he finally agreed to us getting married. I married a nice person, but my former husband had some unresolved issues himself. Neither of us went into the marriage as healthy individuals.

I had no clue that two dysfunctional individuals created the perfect platform for the perfect dysfunctional marriage.

We were both miserable. We made the best of the marriage for as long as we could, but we were both unhappy with ourselves. In fact, we were separated for more time in our eight-year marriage than the time we lived together. The first time we separated was in May 1994, and the final time we separated was January 1999.

Initially, it began with the both of us on the same team, but before long we started to passionately dislike each other. Honestly, to be totally transparent, we should have never married in the first place. We were young, and dysfunctional.

I had major rejection, rebellion, and control issues. These issues permeated all my thoughts, emotions, and decisions. I wanted to fix him, help him, and for us to build a life together.

It was just one problem...ME!

I couldn't get out of my own way! You see; in my desire to fix him, I never saw myself as broken and in need of repair. I was stubborn, super-critical, and I had a serious problem with authority.

The man being the head of the household, in charge of me, and telling

me what to do...screw that! Submission...what is that!? I could NOT submit to the will of God; let alone my husband!

From the very beginning, it was my way or the highway. I never did anything wrong, so I never apologized! Don't get me wrong here, no

marriage ever fails because of one person. This is my story, and I am admitting to the contributions that I made to the destruction of the marriage.

My ex-husband did a lot of things wrong, but he is not telling the story, so I will share my truth. I have learned that by accepting my actions and taking responsibility for my decisions rather than blaming others or acting as a victim is one key to my healing. Several other character defects that aid in the success of my failed marriage were my need to be right, and my inability to forgive.

When he walked out the marital home in 1999, I knew it was for the last time.

 I had become what I called, *"A Throw-Away Wife"*. This was the start of the "*Throw-Away Wife Syndrome" or TAWS*.

Now for the sake of clarity, I will define this syndrome as, *"a complex condition that has identifiable patterns of depression, self-neglect, and emotional baggage that is initiated by the onset of a divorce."* Now this is not a diagnosable condition that you can go to the doctor and get a pill to help heal. *I made up the phrase to describe my inner turmoil.*

Had I initially gone to a medical professional; I am sure that I would have been diagnosed as clinically depressed.

The "*Throw Away Wife Syndrome"* can last indefinitely if effort is not made to identify and address the emotions associated with the death of the marriage. I felt discarded, trampled, depleted, empty, used, abused, and worthless. Oh, and mad as hell! I was furious!

Although, I was the person who filed for the divorce. I was so angry that he didn't fight for our marriage when I had done so much to be a good wife. I had given so much to my ex-husband that I lost myself.

No, wait! I gave so much to my ex-husband that I never learned who I am, or what was most important to me. Now, that is much more accurate.

I was covered with so much garbage, I was an emotional sewer dumping ground before we got married. I heaped onto that emotional dumping ground, his emotional issues, and the complexities of being a wife and mother that there was no opportunity to learn about myself.

My life was a living wasteland.

I filed for divorce in 2001, I spent 1999 to 2001 single just dealing with my issues.

I began to take out the trash, my emotional garbage.

Several of my friends suggested that I date to expedite the healing process.

"The best way to get over one is to replace them."

"Don't chase them, replace them" were common phrases that were given to me at that time. Secretly in my heart I believed we would reconcile.

In the past, when we separated, we would remain sexually active with each other. Sex was safe with my ex-husband, and to be honest it was good! Not only was I still in love with him, but I had a soul tie sexually.

This time, I remained celibate. For the first time since the birth of my children, it felt good to not place myself in a meaningless sexual relationship. I began dating again in 2001 and remarried in 2002. This time I handled the dating and subsequent marriage differently. I married a coworker; we kept our relationship discreet until the wedding invitations were mailed out.

People were shocked! In the beginning of the dating relationship, I was determined not to marry again.

My second, ex-husband (this sounds funny to me) spent a lot of time, and a lot of money wooing me. I felt safe with him for several reasons. First, I knew of his basic character based on our interactions at work. I knew things were different. I was a different person.

My children were teenagers, and I had returned to college. I had learned to value and appreciate myself more. I had done the work to clean up some of the toxicity on the emotional dumping site.

We spent a lot of time talking and getting to know one another. He was a licensed clinical psychologist, he was educated, and I knew his clinical skills were intact. Many of my poor decisions from my past were already different in terms of partner selection.

I had upgraded.

We spent a lot of time having fun, and competing with one another to plan special dates, and other activities. After months of dating I decided to integrate my children into the relationship when it became apparent that we would get married. The four of us dated and went out on so many family excursions. I felt good about my decision to get married, but NOT thoroughly convinced it would be until death do us part.

We married in 2002 and divorced in May 2007. It was strange because we communicated well, but there was a distance between us that was never closed. All these years later, I still don't understand it. I have accepted that some questions will not be answered.

RElate

What areas in the story can you find relatable to your life? Have you ever been married? Have you ever been divorced?

_____

_____

_____

_____

_____

_____

_____

_____

_____

_____

_____

_____

_____

_____

_____

If you are divorced what did you do to contribute to the breakdown of the marriage? Did you accept responsibility for your contributions in order to heal? Divorce is a loss; did you go through the grieving process of the divorce? How long did you grieve?

_____

_____

_____

_____

_____

REcover

As part of the recovery process, did you remain single for a time period to assess your emotional, mental status? Do you embrace the concept that replacing a man with another dating relationship is the best way to heal? Why? Why not? Do you date the same type of men or women? Have you remarried?

_____

_____

_____

_____

_____

_____

_____

_____

_____

_____

_____

_____

_____

_____

_____

_____

_____

R E lease

Acceptance is powerful in the healing process! There are so many unresolved questions left over from my second marriage, but I have learned to accept that I cannot change the outcome. What areas in your life have you come to accept? What areas do you still need to accept in your recovery process?

_____

_____

_____

_____

8 Discounted Self-Worth

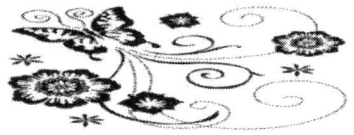

Ladies, is your self-esteem so low that it is priced at or below a value discount coupon? Are you in so much of a need for love, approval, and acceptance that you will allow yourself to be passed around from man to man? Are you constantly giving out free samples of your "Lady Goods" hoping that at some point those free samples will turn into him putting a ring on *it* proposal? Ever gone into a bathroom room and saw an advertisement up in the stall and it had your name and phone number posted?

Are you in a situation that causes you to be the recipient of verbal, emotional, and physical abuse on a regular or repeated basis (even after you were promised that it would never happen again)? If your intimate relationship(s) were compared to that of a business would you be on the verge of receiving a pink slip, being outsourced, downsized, or bankrupt? Speaking of comparing your relationship to a business, are you in a partnership that is inclusive of you and your known partner, or are there "many silent partners?" Does the emotional, financial, or other investments that you have made in the relationship provide you with a rate of return (ROR) worthy of your investment of time and commitment? Are you earning interest, dividends or stock options?

If you answered yes to one or more of these questions, or if your answers left you in a deficit, then you need to increase your value of your self-worth, and self-esteem!

Why would I say that? I can speak from a voice of experience. I have been that woman who placed little to-no-value on myself.

Self-worth is defined as how a person views their own value; confidence in one's own worth or abilities, self-respect or satisfaction in one's self.

There are many ways that we develop confidence or in my case, lack of self-confidence that aids in determining the discount coupon self-worth. Images and subliminal messages can be influenced by family, friends, media, and many other sources. One example that aided in the negative discount coupon value that I placed on myself was a recurring theme of rejection from my peers, and various family members.

This rejection started with the abandonment of my father and continued for many decades until I broke the cycle. Based on research, there is a very distinct difference between self-concept and self-esteem. Self-concept requires reflection on one's self and behavior. Self-esteem is the general attitude about one's self.

So just how do you go from a discounted coupon self-concept to one of value and acceptance?

First, you must acknowledge that you have a poor self-concept. This can be difficult because it requires some honesty, courage, and acceptance. It is NOT an overnight instant process!

My journey took years to be quite honest. If you are looking to learn to love, appreciate and value yourself overnight after discount coupon self-concept, you could be setting yourself up for failure. Frankly, you start valuing yourself with the woman in the mirror. Small steps lead to bigger steps...so start by taking out a mirror.

Find a quiet place, stand in front of a mirror, and just look at yourself. Who do you see staring back at you? What do you like about her? Do you like your hair color? Eye color, cheekbone structure, or your nose?

Sounds easy, right?

Honestly, how many things have you already said that you do not like just within the first five minutes of this exercise? Next, give yourself a nod of approval!

Come on; tell yourself, "I am ok."

Ok, this is major...tell yourself, "I love you_____." Fill your name in the blank line.

You may not be able to do all of this at one time, but I want you to continue the exercise until you are able to tell yourself, "I love you and I value you."

You see, you really are beautiful! You are awesome! You are unique! You are a wonderful, marvelous, beautiful creation!

There is NO ONE else like you. There are seven billion people on this earth and there is NOT another person identical to you! That factor alone is worth celebrating!

Now, if you are anything like me, you are a skeptic and you don't believe me. You may be thinking, *"What makes her an authority?"* I have suffered so much abuse, and mistreatment from possessing a poor self-concept that I got to a place of overflow...all the pain, anger, and rage began to spill out into negative interactions with others. I was hurting and I began to hurt others.

The Big Reveal: Peeling back the layers, and taking off the mask to find me, AND SELF-ACCEPTANCE FINALLY...!

One of the most difficult things for me to do in life has been to accept ME. I know that must sound crazy to some people, but it is true. You see, I suffered from low, fractured, and damaged self-esteem. My self-esteem was like scattered pieces of a tormented spirit. I did not value, or appreciate ME. As a matter of fact, I did not understand that there was a need to accept ME until I was forty years old, and the journey from low self-esteem, and low self-worth continued for another seven years before I reached the plateau of SELF-ACCEPTANCE, FINALLY!

I was 40 years old before I KNEW that I needed to accept me.

Now, I know this sounds impossible, but let us travel back in time so you can get a clearer picture of what I saw in my mirror.

As a child and young adult, I had undergone so much rejection that is was normal to hide behind a mask of pain. Sure, I smiled all the time, but it was a fake painted on smile that hid the flood of tears I cried each night. Often, I did not know or understand the reason for my tears.

No one knew of the rejection, depression and thoughts of suicide that swirled around in my mind. I desired to be loved and accepted so much that I suffered from "people-pleasing syndrome." I would do almost anything just to be accepted by other people. This went on well into my adulthood.

My story is not a sad tale; it is a story of triumph! It is a story of a road traveled by many to self-acceptance. Some people come out on the other side embracing their truth, while others continue to wear the

mask. In my story, I stop wearing the mask and ACCEPT MYSELF...FINALLY!

As a child, I suffered at the hands of men who abused, and molested me. I cried out, but no one saved that little girl starving for protection.

This abuse caused me to create, and wear masks. Ironically, these masks looked like me. When I looked in the mirror, I saw a reflection of myself, but I didn't recognize the person who looked back at me.

I have often said, "I was born with a veil of rejection covering me." Honestly, I believed this, but in order to raise that veil, I needed to remove the mask. I had to understand that man's rejection, that constant, NO was not my final answer.

I rejected myself.

I did not like me.

I was always at a place of disgust with myself.

There were many reasons that I did not like myself. I was the wrong color, the wrong height, too thin, the wrong ethnicity, born in the wrong family, lived in the wrong zip code, in the wrong time zone, in the wrong country, wrong time in history, not smart enough, not pretty enough, wasn't talented enough. Quite frankly, there was always something wrong with me.

I was not born with all these defaults, and deficiencies. I learned to look at myself from a place of deficiency based on the messages that were imposed on me from outside sources. I grew up in the late 70s and 80s. I heard, saw, and read messages that I interpreted as imperfections, but I also had people in my life that reinforced these messages.

This need for acceptance and approval first manifested in the area of education, resulting in my desire to seek approval and acceptance by making good grades in school. I did not desire to make the grade to make the grade, but more to gain the approval of others. In the beginning, I excelled, but I was wearing a mask of success to hide the pain. Education became an easy way for me to gain attention. My need for acceptance and attention lead to the wearing of another mask. This was a layered mask that looked like me, but it developed into a much deeper need for acceptance and approval that would last another thirty years.

As I progressed through middle school, my hormones took over. The attention from boys began to overrule my drive to seek approval from achieving good grades. I started to feel there was no need to work so hard at pleasing others when the size of my hips and the curve of my breast was an easier way to get attention.

By the time I turned twelve years old, I had been a victim of sexual molestation several times, by several men. When I cried out for help, and no one answered by protecting me, I began to understand that even though I was rejected by day, I was desirable at night.

I started to become cognizant of the influence of a woman and the unspoken power she possesses sexually. This sexual awareness became another deep-seated and deep-rooted mask that I would learn to hide behind. If I had some way of peering into the future to gain wisdom of the heartache and pain that would manifest from wearing this mask and my choices that I would make while wearing the mask, I would have spared myself many years of pain.

There was the pain from unwanted pregnancies, multiple abortions, sexually transmitted diseases, date rape, a thoroughfare of sexual escapades, and the repeated cracks, breaks, and tears to my heart from failed relationships, and multiple divorces. The more I desired acceptance, approval, and validation from men via sexual intercourse, the more I experienced rejection, alienation, and heartbreak. I had a warped, twisted definition of love, and sex.

This mask morphed into a serious spiritual problem with fornication. By the time I gave my life over to Christ, I was in such a contaminated state of resentment, bitterness, and retaliation that I had a deep-seated hatred towards men.

I was deceived into believing that my skillset sexually was so good that I could monetize and financially capitalize through prostituting myself. By day, I was a "good girl." At night, I was willing to "play for pay" to the highest bidder, or so I thought!

There is a high price to pay for low living. I realized that I made my first sexual negotiation and deal at the tender age of twelve years old. I am thankful to God that I did not end up on the streets as a prostitute. Lord knows that my life was headed in that direction.

I needed a "vaginal exorcism" ...a cleansing of my soul and all the soul-ties that left me fragmented and broken. I did not look for a priest, rabbi, or pastor to perform this exorcism. No, the only one who could fix this damage was God.

There was just one problem! I thought of God as male...translation, M-A-N! All the men that I had known up until that point had abused me, molested me, and abandoned me.

How or why could I trust God would be any different? The bible references God as the Father...yet, I should trust him? Why?

I had no earthly father to serve as an example...my only examples were on television. They did not look like me, and they certainly did not live in my household!

One day, I caught a glimpse of myself from the inside out. I saw myself spiritually and emotionally. I call it a "solfié" … a soulful self-inventory: I did not like what I saw. I was ugly! This glimpse of the real "me" was far worse than the reflection I saw in the mirror. In fact, after removing layer after layer of the masks, I did not recognize myself. I didn't know what my core values, morals or belief systems were. I did not honor my value system, and I had no idea what values I held sacred. I had no self-esteem, self-value or self-worth.

I discovered that I was so concerned with pleasing other people that I never took the time to cultivate and mature into a person that I valued, validated, or appreciated. I was pitiful, searching for love in all the wrong places, and my life had become the direct results of those bad decisions.

It was during this time I discovered there was a foundation of bitterness, anger, disappointment, and resentment that created a barrier both for me to love and be loved by others. Ironically, LOVE was still the one thing that I desired more than anything. In order to love others, I had to learn to love me…and in order to love me, I needed to learn to accept God's love for me.

Even that was difficult because there is a certain amount of vulnerability necessary in order to give and receive love. I did not trust anyone. My experience showed me it was impossible to trust anyone. As I began to learn about God through His Word, the bible, I began to see myself differently. In fact, I saw most things differently. The cold-hard shell began to break. I went from a place of viewing loving close relationships as a fallacy to understanding that meaningful, loving relationships can occur without drama and dysfunctionalism.

My experience taught me to both run from, and sabotage healthy relationships. Now, I desire to seek peaceful, harmonious relationships. Before, while wearing my mask(s) I didn't mind being controversial, blunt, curt, or sarcastic as I related to others; I now understand none of those behaviors resulted in my need to love others or others loving me. I pushed people away from me and isolated myself by building emotional walls. I did not allow others to get close enough to learn to love me, and I was unable to learn to love others.

Before taking off the mask and letting God transform my heart, I maintained a pompous, critical, condescending attitude toward others. Today, although there are times some of my old UGLY ways of doing things seem more profitable, I am reminded that the seeds I sow today will grow a harvest that I will reap in my future.

It was the Word of God that changed me from the inside out, that renewed, refreshed, and washed me of the old residue of my past and those UGLY masks that I thought hid my pain. Those UGLY masks did not hide my Ugliness from others seeing my ugliness…the masks only hide the ugliness from me seeing the beauty of God radiating from inside of me.

I invite and challenge you to take off your masks to discover the beauty that is being hidden inside of you…it is then that you will discover the real you and learn the true essence of SELF ACCEPTANCE, FINALLY!

RElate

It is difficult for us to see ourselves, and to accept the truth about our imperfections. We usually see ourselves worse than we are or better than what we are. The truth is that we have different personas, or masks that we wear each day.

What masks are you currently wearing to hide your imperfections? Take an honest look at yourself and write your answers below.

_____

_____

_____

_____

R E cover

Recovery always begins with truthfulness and honesty. Now that you have made an assessment of some of your masks (weaknesses, character defects, imperfections, etc.) ask a few people that love you and have your best interest at heart their honest opinion of you? Ok, this may be difficult, but if you want change, it requires honesty and truthfulness. What were the results of your opinion poll? Hint: If different people tell you the same things, there is a big chance that there is some truth to their assessment.

_____

_____

_____

_____

_____

_____

R[lease

Releasing masks is a tricky endeavor. The irony about learning to become transparent is that you only become good at it by practicing being transparent and being transparent is a normally risky. It takes a great deal of vulnerability and a lot of courage.

9 Depression, Suicide, and Chocolate Covered Sedatives

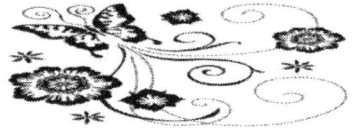

Honestly, this is the most difficult chapter to write! I have written and spoken about my sexual addiction, and have healed by telling my story, and sharing my pain in those areas. However, I have not written or spoke openly about depression, suicide and medication.

As I write…I write afraid of releasing the truth, but I am forging on.

Looking back, I have been clinically depressed for a long time. Some of my symptoms were classic symptoms of depression: depressed mood most of the day, feeling sad, empty and hopeless. I often experienced a marked disinterest in daily activities, unexplained weight loss, or weight gain. Now, I had weight gain, but it could be easily explained. I used food as a source of comfort to help me stuff down those emotions and thoughts that made me feel inadequate, ashamed, guilty and worthless. I was always tired, even though I was always busy doing something. When I was not working two or three jobs, caring for my children, or going to school-I spent much of my time sleeping. It appears sleep was the one thing that I could do to escape my reality that had no negative side effect.

For years, I was on automatic pilot…I did not "feel" my emotions. I just went about my daily affairs without feeling anything. My emotions were turned off which allowed me to function as a "normal" person without being entangled in my confused, angry, deficient and guilty emotions. In fact, most of the decades between my late twenties and my early forties were a comatose state for me emotionally.

I remember the inability to cry. I could not shed a tear for more than ten years. Pain in my life had built up and hardened my inside.

In my thirties, there was an ugly, super darkened pigmented, itchy-scaly rash that appeared on my chest in between my breast one day. I itched like crazy! I went to the dermatologist to have it checked. The doctor biopsied the rash and came back with a super expensive incredibly difficult to pronounce twenty-letter term. I took the medicines and used the creams, but the rash would not go away.

One day, I heard in my spirit, "I will give you a fleshy heart in exchange for the stony-hardened heart."

"What? Lord, what are you trying to tell me?" I asked.

I searched the scriptures and found biblical scriptures in Ezekiel that speak to God replacing my stony heart with a fleshy heart.

I did not understand its meaning.

Not to mention, I was still angry with God!

It had been some years since I prayed more than a superficial prayer. I did not spend time in prayer and communication with Him. He seemed so distant and far away. I had not forgiven God for his disappointing me. I look back now and I laugh. How could I have the audacity to be angry with God, the Creator and the Ruler of all things? Nevertheless, I was!

Since beginning my menstrual cycle at the age of twelve, I have endured years of painful periods with symptoms that include bloating, weight gain, food cravings, cramps, dizziness, fainting spells, vomiting, depression and mood swings. My monthly period has been an unwelcomed interruption for my entire life. In my earlier years, I had more physical symptoms, but as I aged the symptoms became less physical, and more mental and emotional.

In the 1990s it got worse. Every month, I wanted to hide under a rock a few weeks before my period, and after my period things returned to normal. I was diagnosed with Premenstrual Dysphoric Disorder. This is a severe case of PMS. According to the Diagnostic and Statistical Manual of Mental Disorders the Fifth Edition (DSM-5) its symptoms can include:

In the majority of menstrual cycles, at least five symptoms must be present in the final week before the onset of menses, start to improve within a few days after the onset of menses, and become minimal or absent in the week post menses.

Marked affective lability (e.g. mood swings, feeling suddenly sad or tearful, or increased sensitivity to rejection).

Marked irritability or anger or increased interpersonal conflicts.

Marked depressed mood, feelings of hopelessness, or self-deprecating thoughts.

Marked anxiety, tension, and/or feelings of being keyed up or on edge.

Decreased interest in usual activities (e.g. work, school, friends, and hobbies).

Subjective difficulty in concentration.

Lethargy, easy fatigability, marked lack of energy.

Marked change in appetite; overeating; or specific food carvings.

Hypersomnia or insomnia.

A sense of being overwhelmed or out of control.

Physical symptoms such as breast tenderness or swelling, joint or muscle pain, a sensation of "bloating" or weight gain.

I had every single symptom, and at the time I was prescribed Zoloft® as an antidepressant. I didn't understand why I was being given an antidepressant for physical symptoms that occurred monthly, as the result of my period.

I wasn't depressed, and I didn't need medication…I wasn't crazy! I just had an extremely difficult time coping with life when my monthly period interrupted my sense of normal. Looking back, I realized I was depressed, in addition to having these symptoms, I was in a failing marriage; I was employed full-time in a dead-end job that was unfulfilling, and I was struggling financial working a second job. I was not receiving child support; I juggled meeting my financial obligations each month. I wasn't crazy, but I was in denial! This new diagnosis was unbearable, but what would come next took it to a new level!

May 28, 1994, I spoke to my baby brother Lamont for the last time. I was his confidant, his big sister. We shared everything. He was feeling down in the dumps because he had broken up with his girlfriend. My brother was creative, funny, articulate, extremely artistic, a weightlifter, and health buff. He was good at saving money, planning, and achieving his goals.

I will NEVER forget that night…he called me, we talked, I gave my advice, and he listened. I did not listen close enough. I did not hear what he did not say. I did not hear the torment and pain hidden in his heart. There was no way I could have known he would kill himself. I remember hanging up the phone and chuckling that my baby brother is in love. I laughed, not in a sarcastic or evil way; more as if he will be fine…this will pass.

Memorial Day 1994, the Detroit Police contacted my grandmother while we were celebrating the holiday to inform us that the Florida police found my brother dead in his apartment. Based on the estimated timing of death listed on the autopsy, and death certificate…it was shortly after we spoke. Immediately, I knew it was foul play! My brother loved life! It was that evil woman that he was dating. *How could God allow this?*

Guilt immediately settled in and took up residence for more than ten years in my life. *Why didn't I stop it? Why didn't I know the signs? Why didn't I get help? Why didn't I call him back that night? How could I go on living when I knew I was the cause of his death?*

My mind was flooded with questions…

In the chaos, I forgot to shield my six-year-old son from the details of his favorite uncle's death. At six years old, he listened to "He hung himself" repeated several times that day. The shock of those words for me as an adult were traumatic. I cannot comprehend what it was like for my son to hear those words. The days, weeks, months, and years following Lamont's death were a tailspin into years of depression, not only for me, but for my son as well.

The first few days after learning of his death, honestly, I wanted to kill myself! I had so much guilt because I could not be there for him. I wanted to end it all. I knew that was not good, so I went to church to get some help. One of my friends talked with me about

the spirit of suicide being a sneaky and seducing spirit. She was bold and helped me to understand that if I was not careful, and be diligent in prayer, that I would also be a fatality to suicide.

For weeks, I did not bathe, brush my teeth, and comb my hair. All these years later, I still have clothes that I wore for so long the funky body odor could not be removed from my clothes. I didn't have a clue how to handle grief, let alone share with young children about a loved one dying! Maybe, I could've said, *"Uncle Lamont went to heaven. We won't see him anymore right now. Uncle Lamont went to sleep, and he didn't wake up."* I just failed to shield my children from the craziness.

I remember wanting to die! I wanted to be with my brother; feeling as though I had failed him! The guilt was eating me alive! Soon after my brother died, my ex-husband left me too. He left me with two small children that I couldn't care for. I was so angry! I was angry with myself for not preventing this from happening. I was angry at my brother for leaving me. I was angry with the police department for lying on my brother and ruling his death as a suicide rather than a homicide! My brother was a weight trainer, and health nut. He was responsible, he worked daily, paid his bills ahead of time, he didn't drink, smoke, or use drugs. I knew it was a homicide! I was the last person to talk with my brother, and he would NEVER commit suicide! BUT HE DID!

As a matter of fact, the police were contacted by my brother's employer because he missed work, and that NEVER happened! I just knew there was some foul play, no one can convince me otherwise! In my heart all these years later I still want to believe this! Living life after a suicide is difficult at best, and hard at its easiest.

Soon after my brother's death, my son began displaying his emotions, as children often do, by acting out in school! His behavior problems were not in the form of aggression but in severe depression and withdrawal behavior. I couldn't help him (I couldn't help my brother, now I was failing at helping my son) ...so we started grief counseling as a family. I didn't realize how severe we needed to process this traumatic loss! We cried, we talked, we released as much as I could stand it before I ended the therapy for myself. The pain was too deep!

Little did I know ending therapy abruptly was a bad decision! My weight ballooned out of control, but I didn't care. I was living on the edge of "nothing matters," and *"what are we here for?"* I existed by doing only those activities that were absolutely necessary. I had no energy for extras. I even started researching how to commit suicide and make sure my insurance policy paid out to my children. In my mind, I was a failure; worth more dead than alive. I couldn't see past failing my brother, and his death.

The memories of my brother began to fade. I couldn't remember us as children. I couldn't remember how he looked. If someone mentioned him, I would get angry and leave the room. I was numb in my heart and mind for YEARS! I became bitter, crude, mean and critical of others. As long as I was proficient at pointing out deficiencies in others, I didn't have to look at my own! Failing my brother made me feel like a failure in life. It became easy to criticize others rather than deal with my own internal numbness. I wore a mask thinking I was hiding my pain from others, but I was really hiding my truth from myself. Everyone could see I was in emotional pain except me. Family and friends stopped trying to help because I would cut them with sarcasm and inflict severe wounds with my tongue. I didn't mind hurting others. Looking back, I probably enjoyed it.

I wanted to be close to people, but I was so afraid of allowing people to get close to my bleeding heart. The thought of losing people that I loved terrified me! In my mind, it was better to push others away, rather than to allow them to get too close to me and die!

RElate

How are you able to relate to this story about suicide? Write the details of your experience below?

_____

_____

_____

_____

_____

_____

_____

_____

_____

_____

_____

How are you able to relate to feeling depressed? Can you see yourself in the DSM 5 with any of those symptoms?

Please understand the first step to changing a situation is acceptance. I spent too many years in denial, and because I was in denial, I was in pain. It was unnecessary pain. Help was available, but I refused to stop hiding behind the pain! We do not have to continue to suffer from mental illness when so many advances have been made in the field of mental health.

REcover

Recovery after the loss of a love one due to suicide is difficult! Isolation is not a good idea for the survivors. In this section, I list resources for the survivors.

National Suicide Hotline
1-800-273-8255

https://suicideprevention.lifeline.org

Talk to Someone Now - National Suicide Prevention Lifelinehttps://suicidepreventionlifeline.org/talk-to-someone-now/

Suicidehotlines.com

Dialogs: Survivors Postvention Support
810-423-9164
Dialogoinc@gmail.com

Effective Treatment for Mental Illness is available...we don't have to suffer in silence, and we can end the stigma.
1-800-950-NAMI (6264) or **info@nami.org**
National Alliance on Mental Health

Mental Health America

If you or someone you know is in crisis, please call 911, go to the nearest emergency room, call 1-800-273-TALK (8255) to reach a 24-hour crisis center, or text MHA to 741741 at the Crisis Text Line.

10 "I'm in Love With a Man Who Has Never Loved Me"

I am in love with a man who has never loved me.
I am in love with a man who has never loved me!
Have you ever loved someone who doesn't love you?
Let me share my experience, so we can compare our experience…
my every waking moment has been consumed with thoughts of him.
These thoughts possess me both consciously and subconsciously. I
push them out of my cognitive thoughts, but they always return.
I reason and rationalize, how is it possible to love someone who has
never demonstrated any love, affection, or even general humanly
concern for me?
"They" say love is what love does" …that being true, I should have
NO LOVE for him…
During the years, his appearance has changed, as has mine.
As a matter fact, he has taken on many forms of men, but he has
always been the same non-committed, non-attentive, simply not into
me.
If I could count the tears, I have cried,
wondering why he can't, he won't return my affection.
Why he won't acknowledge me, why he won't love me?
What's wrong with me?
Don't I deserve to be loved?
Don't I deserve to be happy? Don't I deserve to be acknowledged?
I have cried this cry for years…. too many years, and I still don't
have answers.
My relationship with him has helped me forge my relationships with
other men.
My involvement with him has taught me to not trust, expect lies, and
expect temporary as an unpleasant fact of life…
I have proven my love for him repeatedly. He has proven his lack of
love for me time and time again…but I remain in love with a man
who doesn't love me.
I am not angry, bitter, or hostile, well NOT ANYMORE.

I have written him, called him, and even hired a private investigator to get him to love me.
For me to heal from my sickness of poor companion selection, I must get over my love affair with HIM.

I am not desperate, lonely, or dysfunctional...well, no more that the next person. I stand before you transparent, human. Just seeking love and acceptance.... you see this man that I am in love with...I carry his DNA inside of me.

He is with me all the time...I can't escape him, for I am his legacy...I am him and he is I.
This mystery man is my father...and I love him,

I just wish, hope, and pray,
one day he will love me.

The End is Only the beginning...

Made in the USA
Columbia, SC
05 July 2020